THE BEST OF **HEALTH**

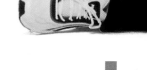

The Best

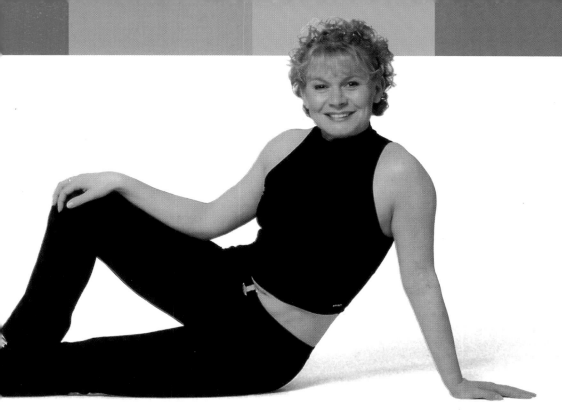

# of Health

Looking good and feeling fit

GLENDA McKAY

GRANADA
MEDIA

First published in Great Britain in 2000 by Granada Media

an imprint of Andre Deutsch Limited in association with Granada Media
Group
76 Dean Street
London W1V 5HA

10 9 8 7 6 5 4 3 2 1

A catalogue record for this book is available from the British Library

ISBN 0 233 99733 4

The publisher wishes to thank Karen Sullivan for her contribution

Cover and page design by Roger Hammond
Reprographics by Jade Reprographics
Printed and bound in Italy by Officine Grafiche DeAgostini

Contents

Introduction

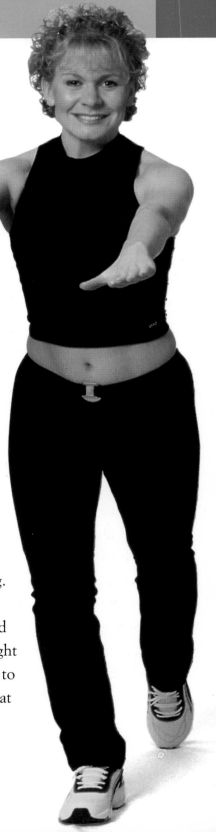

HELLO, I'M GLENDA MCKAY and I am proud to introduce to you my first book, *The Best Of Health*. As the title suggests, this book is your step-by-step guide to a healthier, happier life.

Be fit, look stylish, eat well and feel relaxed – wouldn't we all like to achieve these goals? Well, we can, and it doesn't have to be a drag, or completely rule your life. By reading *The Best of Health* you will learn how to take charge of your life NOW and change it for the better! This book gives you all the knowledge you need to improve your diet, fitness, wardrobe, beauty routine and stress levels,

Don't worry, I am not going to ask the impossible of you. The last thing I want to do is encourage people to get obsessive about anything. Life (and I know this sounds boring) is all about MODERATION. Now, I am not going to pretend to be some angelic figure who never has a late night or a glass or two of wine. What I am going to try to illustrate is that you can have fun and be healthy at the same time.

This book aims to show you ways of adopting a new lifestyle which is easy to follow without having to spend six hours a day in the gym and only eating celery. Each chapter deals with a separate topic, ranging from nutrition to image and self-belief, exercise to rest and relaxation, and alternative therapies to beauty treatments. It's a mass of knowledge all about how to make YOU feel better within YOU.

I was inspired to write this book because there is such a lot of confusion and bad education when it comes to health issues these days. We don't understand how much exercise a week is good for us or how much rest we should be getting, how much fat we should be avoiding a day or what types of fat are essential in our diet. Also, if we get disillusioned with our GPs, what alternative therapies are available and which one is best for a particular ailment? It really is a minefield out there and I thought it was about time that this was addressed in a simple, easy-to-follow book.

I am sure you will enjoy reading *The Best of Health* from cover to cover and I can guarantee that, once it's in your life, it will keep on reappearing as you use it for reference in years to come.

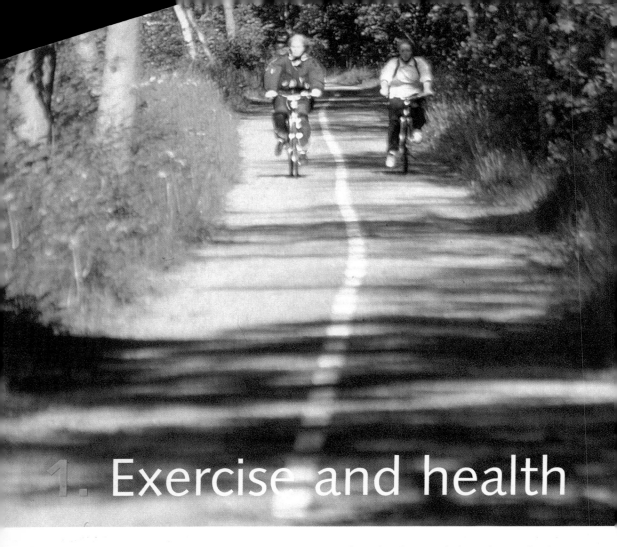

1. Exercise and health

FOR MANY OF us, the very word exercise produces a cold sweat. And to be fair, until recently, exercise had a fairly grim reputation. It was essential to weight-loss (and anything associated with that couldn't be fun), and apart from jogging or the standard aerobic class, there wasn't a lot on offer.

That's all changed. There are literally dozens of types of exercise now available. If you like sweating it out in a gym, you have dozens to choose from; you may enjoy yoga, pilates, step, body conditioning or aquarobics (exercise in water). Swimming may be your scene, or you might just enjoy kicking a football around in the park with a few friends. With exercise, anything goes. The secret is to find something that raises the heart-rate, involves the use of muscles, keeps you fit and makes you feel good. Even brisk walking, three times a week, can have that benefit, so you don't need to don a leotard or a designer tank top to get your body moving. What's more, everyone is doing it – exercise has become positively fashionable.

Most people I speak to say they haven't got time to exercise and I understand how they feel. That's why I decided to create an aerobics video which even the busiest working mum can use and see the results.

Fit, Fresh and Funky has different colour coded sections each lasting seven minutes, and each with slightly different themes. You must always start with the yellow zone to warm up gently and stretch your muscles, then you can fast forward until you see the workout that you fancy that day. You can mix and match your workout – for example, picking the high energy zone followed by slinky hips and toned thighs. If you are in a rush to pick up the kids from school, just do the yellow zone – I guarantee you'll feel better and fitter after those seven minutes alone. If you have time and feel like Wonder Woman one day, you can do all seven sections and have the ultimate workout. Your routine is unique to you, tailored to fit how you feel that day, so you'll never get bored of being fit, fresh and funky.

SO WHY IS EXERCISE IMPORTANT?

Exercise is good for both the body and the mind. Physically, regular exercise helps to develop muscle tone and strength, and to control weight. Besides strengthening the muscles, including the heart, regular exercise is believed to make bones stronger by increasing the amount of calcium they absorb. It has also been shown to reduce high blood pressure and cholesterol levels. Psychologically, regular exercise helps contribute to a feeling of well-being, as well as relieving the effects of stress.

People who exercise regularly are more likely to continue to exercise throughout their lives. As people age, the benefits of regular exercise grow more important. While genetics plays a role in the effects of ageing, exercise has a beneficial effect on the ageing body, helping to maintain fitness and slow down the physical effects of growing old.

The body becomes deconditioned with age and, if not properly exercised, can develop significant problems in the muscles, bones, and heart and lungs. Muscles wither and lose their tone, leading to more frequent tearing of muscles and tendons. Bones become weak and brittle, fracturing more easily and more often. The cardiovascular (heart and lung) system adjusts down to the point where any little chore can cause an increase in pulse rate and blood pressure and earlier development of

Sheree Murphy
✿ *Try to pick a type of exercise that doesn't bore you otherwise, like me, you will give up fast on it. I like to swim, as it is not pounding at my joints like aerobics or running would.*

atherosclerosis (congestion of the arteries).

If you get no exercise, you lose muscle tissue. Apart from anything else, this puts your skeleton under serious strain, as muscles are part of the fabric that holds the body upright. Muscle burns fat. If you don't have any muscle, you will be using less and less fat, and laying down more in stored deposits. Your heart will be under strain. You will probably suffer from niggling health complaints, like headaches, insomnia, digestive problems and skin disorders. Why? Because exercise keeps things ticking over in your body. When you are fit, your body works at optimum level. When you are not, things begin to slide and one by one your body systems start to give up the ghost. Every organ, every cell in our bodies, needs oxygen to carry out its function. If you don't get enough exercise, your heart has to work doubly hard to get oxygenated blood around the body. Sometimes the supply is just not adequate enough, and your body goes into retreat.

If that's not reason enough, when you find an activity that you enjoy doing, exercise helps to ensure good, restful sleep, keeps you supple, increases your confidence, gives you much, much more energy and adds a great deal of pleasure to your life.

It's pretty clear your present and future health depends on you getting some exercise. Why not start now?

WHAT KIND OF EXERCISE?

Exercise programmes can be designed to develop one or a number of aspects of our fitness. For example, there is fitness for cardiovascular efficiency, for strength, speed, flexibility, muscle endurance, power, agility and balance.

AEROBICS

For an exercise to be aerobic it must increase your intake of oxygen. Walking, running, biking and swimming can easily fit the bill – as can a good game of football in the park. A major benefit of aerobic conditioning is its effect on your heart and lungs. Evidence shows that aerobic exercise helps decrease the risk of cardiovascular disease, the number-one killer of both men and women in the West. It helps to lower your risk of heart disease by strengthening the heart and making it more efficient. When you exercise, your muscles require more fuel – oxygen. So your heart pumps harder in order to push more blood, which transports the oxygen to the muscles. When the heart works harder on a regular basis, it grows stronger and more efficient.

If you are feeling stressed out, the best cure is exercise. I always find that if I have a problem when I go out for a run it's halved by the time I return and as a bonus I feel energized and positive. This is as a result of endorphins (feel-good chemicals produced by the brain) being released into my bloodstream.

Aerobic exercise can also make you feel younger by boosting your self-esteem. You feel more control over your environment and benefit from the positive feedback from friends you exercise with, as well as improved muscle strength and gains in aerobic fitness level. It can also improve your mental attitude. A study of 26 university athletes found that a 30-minute session of riding a special exercise cycle reduced anxiety significantly, and that the effect continued for as long as an hour after the aerobic session.

Aerobic exercise also helps to increase your metabolism – the rate at which your body burns calories. When your heart is working hard, you burn enough calories to reduce body fat, leading to weight loss It is also effective in helping to maintain your strength as well.

When undertaking aerobic exercise, consider the following guidelines:

■ The session must have a genuine aerobic component that lasts for a minimum of 20 minutes at an intensity measured preferably for a minimum heart rate of 120 bpm (see page 12).

■ Exercise should take place at least three times a week.

■ At least 5 minutes must be spent performing a range of stretching and warming up exercises at the start, and slow stretching and cooling down at the end

■ Take your time moving from the warm-up to the actual aerobic exercise

AEROBIC EXERCISE CAN INCLUDE:

● **Walking briskly**	● **Skipping**	● **Tennis**
● **Swimming**	● **Circuit training**	● **Squash**
● **Ice-skating**	(undertaking a	● **Badminton**
● **Rollerblading**	variety of	And virtually any
● **Aerobics classes**	different types of	other form of
● **Aquarobics**	exercise one after	activity that
● **Dancing**	the other)	raises your heart
● **Team sports**	● **Climbing**	rate to its target
● **Jogging**	● **Rowing**	level (see page 12)
● **Running**	● **Cycling**	and keeps it there
	● **Skiing**	for at least 20 minutes.

FLEXIBILITY

Flexibility refers to a range of motion or movement of a joint or a group of joints. In most people, joints have the potential to move through a greater range of motion than the muscles that surround them will allow. Through regular stretching, the muscles' capacity to extend fully is increased, thus allowing the joint a greater range of movement.

Without regular stretching, muscles tend to lose flexibility, so that when they are called upon to perform an extreme movement (such as running for a bus, or lifting something), they are less able to extend to their full range of movement, resulting in damage and injury.

Therefore, stretching:

■ prevents injuries

■ increases the range of movement of the muscles

■ improves co-ordination

■ improves relaxation of the muscles

■ prevents muscles tightening after movement (stiffness!)

When you are stretching, take the following guidelines into consideration:

■ Avoid bouncing, jerky movements.

■ Stretching should be regular – say, three to four times a week. Noticeable changes occur within two to three weeks.

■ Breathe slowly, deeply and evenly.

■ Do not stretch to the point where breathing is strained.

- Do not overstretch. Go to the point where the stretch is felt but is not painful.
- Hold the stretch in a comfortable position.
- Stretch only when your muscles are warm.
- Concentrate on relaxing the areas being stretched.
- Hold each stretch for 15 to 30 seconds and if possible even longer.

WEIGHT TRAINING

Weight training or resistance training is usually considered a pastime for bodybuilders and athletes who wish to pump iron for muscle bulk. However, everyone can benefit from some weight training, and here's why:

- Weight training helps to develop muscular strength and endurance
- It helps to increase the amount of muscle in the body.
- It improves posture.
- It tones up the overall look of the body.
- It can help to rehabilitate muscles that have been injured, or rarely used.
- It helps prevent the loss of muscle that occurs with age.
- It increases your metabolism (muscles burn fat!)

The idea is to use weights, either on a machine or free-standing, to perform a series of repetitions that work specific muscle groups. If you stretch before and after training, and don't work your muscles beyond the point that your fitness instructor suggests, you will not end up with bulging muscles (unless, of course, you want them). Weight training is not aerobic, so it does virtually nothing for your cardiovascular

system. What it does do is condition and tone your muscles so that they work more efficiently – and burn up fat. The result of consistent weight training is a lean body.

Consider the following guidelines when undertaking a weight training programme:

- Use a weight that is appropriate for your level of fitness. You'll need an instructor to help you with this.
- For the first two to four weeks, do only one set of eight to 12 repetitions for each exercise.
- After that, perform two to three sets of eight to 12 repetitions for each exercise in every work out. When more than 12 repetitions can be completed in the final set, increase the weight used by about two per cent.
- Exercise three days each week with a rest day in between each workout.
- Warm up at least five minutes before lifting weights. This includes stretching and loosening up exercises, and maybe a three- to four-minute stint on the exercise bike – to get really warm. If your body is not warm and stretched, you are very likely to strain or even tear a muscle.
- Pay special attention to safety. An instructor will help you assess whether or not you have any weaknesses, and help you to perform exercises at a level that is appropriate for you.
- Take time to stretch and cool down following the session.

BODY CONDITIONING

Body conditioning is a great way to isolate muscle groups and tone them, making them stronger, longer and leaner. Two sections of *Fit, Fresh and Funky* concentrate on conditioning: slinky hips and toned thighs, and firm bums and flat tums. In these workouts we do slow, controlled exercises with lots of repetition to get your body looking really good.

EXERCISE BASICS

- While you might feel great in specially designed sports gear, it's not a must. Clothing should be comfortable and unrestricting, but apart from that, anything

Steve Magan

✿ *Watch out, all you guys heading towards your thirties! I definitely noticed my metabolism slowing down and realized that a little exercise would keep those extra pounds from piling on.*

✿ *If you exercise you will look fresher, your skin will glow, your mood will lift and your eyes will sparkle. This is due to the endorphins released into your bloodstream whilst exercising.*

goes. Some of the tighter, lycra kits have advantages in that they do not hamper movement in any way, and their fabric is designed to 'breathe' to avoid overheating. If this kind of outfit isn't for you, stick with a cotton T-shirt and whatever feels most comfortable on the bottom half.

- Shoes are crucial. Choose a pair of running shoes (trainers), to absorb stress on the feet. They should have a thick, layered sole that runs the length of the shoe, with a soft inner cushion and tough outer layer. Shoes should be flexible enough to allow your feet to bend, but also provide some support. Most importantly, they should be comfortable.
- Wear a pair of cotton socks (which allow your feet to breathe) with your shoes at all times. This will help to prevent chafing and blisters.
- Carry a good supply of liquid. Water is best, and lukewarm is better than cold, which can cause a spasm in the digestive tract if you drink it when you are very, very hot. As a rule of thumb, drink two glasses of fluid 15 to 20 minutes before heavy exercise and one glass at 15 to 20 minute intervals throughout. Continue drinking after exercise to keep your body hydrated. When I was training for the London Marathon I actually had to practise drinking to get used to taking on fluid as I ran and not developing a stitch. It is crucial to drink as often as you can in an endurance event such as that, as you are dehydrating so fast and if the liquid is not replaced you can get serious cramp.
- It is best to leave at least an hour after eating before exercise, as you can develop a serious stitch if your food is still digesting when you start. Also you need the digested fuel ready in your body to power your muscles for the optimum workout.
- Warm up. Begin by running a short distance at a slow speed, to warm the muscles. This makes them less resistant to exercise, and helps to prevent injuries.
- Stretch. When your muscles are warm, perform a series of stretching exercises. This loosens the muscles in preparation for exercise, and can help to prevent injuries

and stiffness later. Warming up and stretching should make up about 10 per cent of your exercise time. Pay particular attention to the muscles that you will be using in your primary exercise.

- Cool down. A cool down period is a vital part of an exercise session. This involves gradually decreasing the intensity of the exercise until the body returns to its 'resting' state. Perform some all-over gentle stretches. This helps the muscles of the body return blood to the heart rather than allowing it to pool in the muscles, which causes stiffness.
- Work up to exercising at an increased intensity. Any change in activity level should be gradual, not sudden.
- Use your heart rate as a guide to the intensity of exercise.

TAKING YOUR PULSE

Your pulse acts as a guide to your heart rate. It should be monitored periodically during an exercise session, and you can adjust the intensity of your exercise to bring your heart rate to the recommended level. The recommended heart rate level is called the target heart rate.

Your theoretical maximum heart rate is 220 minus your age (so if you were thirty, for instance, it would be 190). To be gaining cardiovascular improvements from your exercise your heart rate should be 60-90% of the maximum figure, depending on how fit you are.

You can work out your range like this:

220 – your age x 0.9 = your upper level
220 – your age x 0.6 = your lower level

CHECK FOR A PULSE

- On the thumb side of the wrist, about 1.5 cm above the wrist crease and about 1.5 cm in from the side of the wrist.
- At the carotid arteries in the neck, which run up either side of the Adam's apple, in the hollow between the Adam's apple and the neck muscle.

Check your pulse by pressing two fingers on either of the pulse points (not both). **Never use**

your thumb to take a pulse since it has a pulse of its own.

If you do not feel something immediately, press a little deeper and move your fingers around gently to find the pulse point.

The pulse can be taken for six seconds (and multiplied by ten), for ten seconds (and multiplied by six) or for 15 seconds (and multiplied by four) to get the number of beats per minute.

Check your target heart-rate zone and make sure you keep within it, both for safety and for best results.

HOW MUCH EXERCISE DO WE NEED?

Surprisingly, our exercise needs change little as we age. Children require – and normally get – as much exercise as adults. We should all aim to get at least 20 to 30 minutes' exercise, three or four times a week. That exercise should involve raising the heart rate to its target level (see above). If you find it difficult to take a pulse, try the 'talk test'. If you cannot comfortably talk (or whistle) while exercising, you are probably working too hard.

If you haven't exercised in a while, you'll need to take it easy to begin with. It normally takes two to three weeks for your body to adapt to the new requirements made upon it.

Once you get going, there will be no stopping you building up your routine as high as you like. Always make sure you give your body at least two days a week rest though. When I was training for the marathon I would run over 50 miles a week and this had to be spread over five days. The two rest days were essential for my muscles to recover and repair. Also, if I overtrained, my body's immunity would decrease and I would become lethargic and probably come down with a virus, and then I wouldn't be able to train at all.

Freya Copeland
✿ *Three times a week to the gym for a cardio-vascular workout, plus a little resistance training, keeps me feeling fit and has definitely helped me reduce my weight. I used to be about two dress sizes bigger than I am now and simply by working out I have slimmed off and toned up without going on a starvation diet.*

HOW TO INCLUDE EXERCISE IN A BUSY LIFE

There's no question that exercise can be pretty low down a list of priorities. When you spend your life rushing from one thing to the next, and have only enough energy to flop in front of the television in the evenings, it's difficult to imagine when you could possibly fit it in.

First and foremost, remember that exercise is something for *you*. It will make you feel good, it will give you energy and it will give you confidence. Taking time to do something that is entirely selfish is incredibly healthy. It's your block of time, and you can create it if you really want to. When you exercise, you sleep better and you'll find you need less sleep. According to some studies, you'll need about an hour less a night, if you are fit. Call that hour your exercise time for three or four days a week, and on the other days do with it what you will.

You always have time for the things you put first. Make exercise a priority. Put it at the top of your list. Make a date with yourself, write it in your diary, and don't break it. If you can't manage exercise after work, try lunchtimes. If that's impossible, try setting your alarm for an hour earlier. It's difficult to get out of bed the first few times, but once you've settled into a routine it will become easier and easier. Early morning exercise is a great way to start the day – you'll feel energized and your mind will be more focused.

Exercise need not mean a visit to the gym. A long, brisk walk is equally effective. If you've got kids and you can't get away, take them with you. Play football in the park with your children at the weekends – a good hour of chasing a ball is about as aerobic as it gets. You don't need to choose the same sort of exercise every time. Be imaginative. Meet up with a friend in the park in the early evening and rollerblade. Or hire a bike and explore the neighbourhood. Join a step class or an aquarobics class. Try dry-slope skiing. Anything you can do will make a difference.

Many offices have gyms near by. If the thought leaves you cold, go and investigate. Chances are they have all kinds of classes, from spinning on bikes to pilates. Find one that suits you and make that a once-a-week date. Even if you only manage a swim every now and then, it's a step in the right direction.

If you work at home, try climbing the stairs for 20 minutes. Throw on your favourite exercise video. *Fit, Fresh and Funky* can give you a seven-minute fix of fun fitness – and I don't believe that you haven't got seven minutes to spare. Do it while the baby's asleep in the afternoon! Mix and match the sections that you do and you will soon feel fitter. Take a quick walk to the shops for your papers, rather than driving. Run for the bus. Take the stairs instead of the lift. Find ways to move your body, even if it means dancing in the kitchen while you cook! Explain to your friends what you are doing, and set up a series of dates to learn, say, badminton or squash, or meet up for a game of tennis or just a quick run in the park. Exercise can be incredibly sociable, and there's no reason why you shouldn't join up with friends to do it. Leave your car halfway on the school run, or your daily commute, so that you are forced to walk (quickly!) for half your journey. If you want to do it, if you make it a priority, you'll make the time for exercise.

Exercise	Weight control	Sleep	Digestion	Cardiovascular endurance	Approximate energy used per minute (calories)
Walking	8	6	5	6	5-7
Jogging	10	8	6	10	12-16
Swimming	5	8	7	10	6-11
Cycling	9	8	6	10	8-15
Tennis	6	5	6	7	5-11
Golf	3	3	5	4	5-8
Surfing	6	8	7	10	6-11
Skiing (downhill)	5	8	6	6	6-10
Skipping/Jumping	7	5	5	7	5-11
Step classes	8	7	7	9	9-14
Aerobics	8	7	7	9	9-14
Handball/Squash	8	6	7	10	10-15

Malandra Burrows
✿ *Exercise is therapeutic, if you go out for a run or for a swim with a big problem in your mind, by the time you get back, it won't seem half as bad. Get exercising!*

WHICH EXERCISE WHEN?
Aerobic exercise is likely to make you feel invigorated, so it's probably not the best choice for a late-evening activity. Try to avoid aerobics up to two hours before bedtime (unless, of course, you are dancing the night away).

Suitable late-night activities might include some yoga (see page 50), some simple stretching, or some spot exercises. Try the purple or green sections of *Fit, Fresh and Funky*. They concentrate on specific muscle groups, toning and strengthening them without raising the heart rate so much that you won't be able to sleep.

The type of exercise you choose depends on why you are doing it. All of us should take some aerobic exercise several times a week for the good of our hearts and lungs, not to mention overall health. But there are other reasons for exercise, and there are plenty of different ways to achieve fitness, relaxation and conditioning.

If you want to lose weight, you need exercises that burn fat. Any of the aerobic exercises do this, as does weight training. When you build up muscle, your body becomes a fat-burning machine. Muscle burns fat and if you are overweight, chances are you don't have enough of the less wobbly bits.

If you want to relax, try one of the martial arts, like T'ai chi. Yoga is excellent for relaxation and flexibility, and you will become fit, albeit at a slower rate. Swimming and team sports, where you meet up with a group of interesting people, can be enormously relaxing, especially if you make it fun.

If you just want to feel better, try to incorporate exercises that offer a bit of all of the above. The key to implementing a successful exercise routine is to make it fun. If you enjoy what you are doing, you are more likely to continue. Once you start to feel the benefits, you'll be hooked.

The table opposite gives you an idea of the various benefits of some of the most popular types of exercise. Scores are rated out of 10.

WALKING FOR HEALTH

Brisk walking is one of the most efficient and easiest forms of exercise, and one of the best ways to improve general health and lung capacity. Like all exercise it will make you fit and healthy, prevent illness, allow relaxation which will reduce stress levels, and help your body to deal with common ailments.

■ Walking is an aerobic exercise which uses a great deal of energy and increases your heart rate. This strengthens the heart so that it pumps more efficiently, and improves the health of your heart and circulatory system, as well as your lungs. Walking quickly, you will burn up more calories per minute than in most other sports while expending less effort.

■ Walking has become particularly popular because almost anyone can participate, and it can be done alone or with someone else. I love walking and get out into the beautiful Yorkshire Dales as often as I can with my parents. They introduced me to walking for pleasure as soon as I could do it and you only need to look at how healthy and toned my mum is on the video to see how it can benefit you. It doesn't cost anything and you get your lungs full of wonderful fresh, clean air.

■ Research has found that a brisk 30-minute walk at least three times a week helps to reduce the rate of bone loss in post-menopausal women. Walking is weight-bearing exercise, which helps to build bone mass, and keep your heart healthy. Even if you suffer from osteoporosis, walking is one of the safest exercises you can undertake.

■ A ten-minute walk modifies your mood,

EXERCISE ON THE SPOT

EXERCISE BIKES

Exercise bikes are normally stationary, although riding an ordinary bike will have the same effect. Bikes can contribute an aerobic component to an exercise programme. They can also be used for warming up and cooling down, and for this reason alone they are useful. They can improve general fitness, leg strength, and mobility in the knees and hips. They can reduce body fat and are especially useful for the obese or arthritic, because they help support body weight. If you've got some money to spare and exercising out of the house isn't your scene, an exercise bike might be a good investment – as long as you use it!

TREADMILLS

An alternative to stationary cycling is stationary walking or jogging. Treadmill walking or running offers a good form of cardiovascular conditioning and can help burn up body fat. As with exercise bikes, the main disadvantage of treadmills is the problem of maintaining motivation. They are useful for people who don't like running outdoors, or in poor weather, and they are great for the warm-up and cool-down phases of exercises in an indoor setting. They do not, however, hold any other advantage over outdoor jogging. I have used treadmills when it is snowing outside and slippery underfoot. There really is no substitute for outdoor training though. It is so much more demanding but so much more fun – at least the view changes.

ROWING MACHINES

Rowing is an excellent form of aerobic exercise. It has an added advantage over running and cycling in that it uses the upper body and therefore increases the work effort and can contribute to upper body strength. Motivation, again, can be a problem because anyone but an experienced rower will find that the novelty wears off pretty quickly.

SKIPPING ROPES

Skipping is a great exercise in that it's aerobic, uses both upper and lower body muscles and it helps to improve co-ordination. It can, however, be difficult to maintain for the required 20 to 30 minutes, and it can be fairly tedious in the long run. More exercise is expended in jogging than in skipping, largely because the energy requirement of an activity is dependent on the amount of muscle involved. Jogging apparently uses more muscles than skipping in place. Nevertheless, it's a good way to warm up and cool down, and if you have children, skipping is a great way to get some exercise together.

BURNING FAT, BURNING CALORIES

On page 17 we discuss the best exercises for weight control. Check the list to see if your favourite exercise appears there. To burn fat, you need muscle. To create muscle tissue, you need to exercise. It's as simple as that.

The notion that lower-intensity exercises such as walking and jogging are best for fat-burning simply isn't true. It is true that the proportion of fat to carbohydrate burned is greater with low-intensity exercise. Yet higher-intensity exercise such as brisk running (or cycling) expends more total calories. More to the point, the absolute number of fat calories expended is also greater.

That said, even very high-intensity exercises (sprinting, for example) that burn carbohydrates almost exclusively will still enable you to burn body fat. That's because when exercise ends and the muscles start recovering, fat-burning kicks in as the muscles use incoming carbohydrates for rebuilding glycogen stores.

Another reason exercise boosts fat-burning is because your muscles become 'trained' over time to use more fat as fuel. What happens is that regular exercise increases the activity of certain muscle enzymes that play a role in fat-burning. This spares muscle glycogen and improves endurance. Further, since exercise – particularly strength-training exercise – increases muscle mass, more calories get burned simply because there is more muscle mass to support. This makes it easier to control your weight.

OVER-EXERCISE

Let's look at the other side of the coin. What about fitness freaks? You know the type: they head for the gym at every available moment, can be found doing press-ups at ungodly hours of the day, and hit the cycling track in even the most torrential downpour. Exercise is great – and the more you get, the better. To a point. Over-exercise can be dangerous, and it can be addictive. When you exercise, you experience a high from special chemicals called endorphins that are released into your bloodstream. These are effectively the body's own feel-good drugs and they are one of the reasons why exercise is so rewarding, and has the ability to lift your mood. Some people get accustomed to this feeling, and can't function without it.

So why is over-exercise dangerous? For one thing, it can put too much pressure on your heart, which has to work incredibly hard to keep up with your pace. Secondly, you run the risk of becoming too thin, which can play havoc with your hormones if you are a woman (causing infertility or a cessation of periods, for example). You can exhaust resources that are required to keep your body functioning, and it's absolutely essential that you get plenty of extra nutrients to keep things going. Chances are that you won't manage it. Many athletes suffer from nutritional deficiencies because they use up so many extra nutrients when they train.

So find a balance. That's what we aim for in all aspects of life. Everything in moderation, and you'll look good and feel great.

which quickly raises energy levels and keeps them high for up to two hours.

- A walk can counteract the fatigue you normally feel after a big meal. Digesting large meals increases the blood and oxygen flow to the digestive system, which draws energy away from the muscles and brain, making you tired and fuzzy-headed. A walk will ensure that blood and oxygen circulate throughout your body.

- Walking can provide pain relief by releasing endorphins, which are the body's natural pain-killers. You'll need to walk for at least 20 minutes each day to experience the benefits.

- Walking, like other aerobic exercise, such as swimming and biking, strengthens your whole body. Walking conditions the muscles of the buttocks, legs, back and abdomen, which encourages better posture and protects the back.

- Walking can also act as a form of relaxation. Concentrate on your steps as you move, counting out loud to keep up the rhythm, and you will soon achieve the same effects as a relaxation programme, which gives the brain a chance to rejuvenate and allows adrenaline, which runs through your body in excess when you are stressed, to subside. The important thing is to concentrate while you are walking, and allow your mind to clear. If you find yourself thinking about problems, make a conscious attempt to concentrate on counting. Exercising for 35 to 40 minutes each day can both produce feelings of euphoria associated with endorphins, and reduce the ill-effects of stress, which include headaches, nausea, aches and pains, insomnia, fatigue and digestive disorders.

■ Every weight-loss study in existence offers evidence that people who exercise regularly lose more weight and keep it off. Even 20 minutes, three times a week can help to burn off calories. Walking just one mile (1.5km) will burn up about 100 calories. So if you walk for 30 minutes daily at a fairly brisk pace, you will easily burn up about 1,000 calories in a week. If you walk for an hour at the same pace, you can burn up 2,000 calories. And apart from the high rate of calories burned, you will be creating muscle with which to burn even more – a higher muscle bulk means a higher metabolism, which means you'll burn off calories even faster as time goes on. Furthermore, walking releases endorphins, which make you feel great and suppress hunger. After a long walk you'll feel less hungry and full of energy.

ACTIVELY LOSING WEIGHT

You need to burn 3,500 calories to lose just one pound of fat. Consider how your daily activities tot up.

Activity	Calories burnt per hour	Activity	Calories burnt per hour
Sports		disco dancing	400
aerobics	430	gardening (digging)	480
circuit training	510	gardening (general)	250
running	400		
squash (competition level)	840	**Housework**	
swimming		floor scrubbing	400
(competition level)	600	ironing	200
swimming (relaxed)	400	polishing	200
jogging	300	vacuuming	250
cycling (competition level)	660		
		Daily Activities	
Hobbies		climbing stairs	660
cycling (relaxed)	240	strolling	240
walking briskly	360	watching television	100
dancing	350	sitting at a computer	100

If you are the type of person who chooses the lift over the staircase, consider the fact that you'll burn about ten calories standing there. Use the stairs, and you've used up over 100. Run up the stairs instead of walking and you'll burn an extra 30 or 40 calories. Try to be more active, even when you're not:

■ When walking, do it actively, using good posture and full breathing. This will turn even a short stroll into an aerobic activity.

■ While standing in a queue, practise your posture. This uses up more energy than just slouching.

■ Every time you look up at your computer screen or across the office, accompany the action with the sliding back of your shoulder blades to allow you to take a deep breath.

■ Watching television in the evening, sit properly in your chair and practise the breathing exercise. This will also help you digest dinner.

■ Going round the supermarket, use the trolley as a prop to help you bring your body into a more upright position. This means you will be using your muscles more fully and even has a slight weight-training effect – which you can increase by using a couple of baskets if your shop is not too large.

■ Although each individual effort may only take a couple of minutes, by the end of the day they can add up to the equivalent of a formal 30- or 40-minute aerobic exercise session without you even noticing.

Exercise can be enjoyed by everyone, whatever age you are. You can be competitive by taking up a new sport such as tennis or squash, be inspired by learning a new skill like Yoga or pilates, push yourself to the limit by entering a long distance running race or even combat your fears by taking up rock climbing. The list is endless and there's no doubt you'll have fun, and what could be better than that – having fun and getting healthy! Go on! What's stopping you?

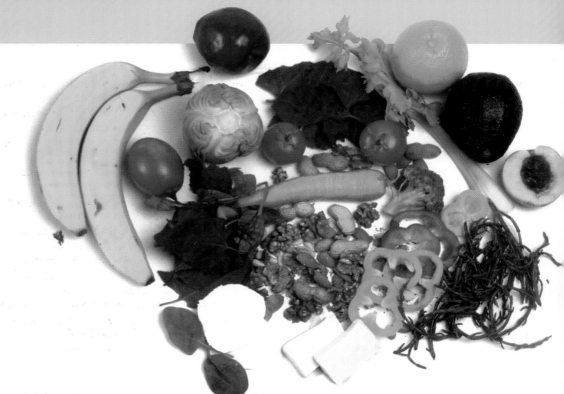

2. Fabulous food

WE ARE SURROUNDED by food. Never before have we had such variety, so many ways to cook it, so many restaurants, fast-food outlets, ready-made meals, such enormous supermarkets. And, as a nation, we are undoubtedly getting fatter, which means that we are eating the stuff. But, weirdly, we have also embarked on a kind of love-hate relationship with food. We eat too much of it, but food has become the enemy. We fill our plates with fattening foods, pick up a burger on the way home from work, eat chocolate bars and bags of crisps, and still find room for a ready-made meal. Our lives are so busy that we eat quickly and rarely notice what we are eating. It's no wonder we are getting fat. We love to eat, but we do it on the run, we eat more than we should because we haven't eaten properly all day, and then we feel guilty and impose a starvation diet the next day.

It's time to stop the roller-coaster ride. There are so many wonderful, fresh and delicious foods now available and, best of all, we have learnt different ways to cook them: choose Indian, Thai, Italian, Chinese, American, Greek – you name it. No time, I can hear you murmur. Wrong! You can cook a full chicken dinner inside 25 minutes if you have the ingredients on hand. You can cook a fresh pasta dish in less than ten. You can grab a cup of home-made, pre-prepared soup from the fridge and, with a salad and a wholegrain bread roll, you've got a meal in five minutes flat.

We all know people who look healthy and seem to live on a packet of fags and endless cups of coffee. There are thin people who exist on chocolate, Diet Coke and crisps. They may look great now, but I can guarantee you that they won't in a few years' time. Our bodies are comprised of the elements of our food – in other words, we are, very literally, made up of what we eat. Sure you can choose quick-to-prepare ready meals and burgers. Yes, they will provide energy to live on, but they also contain toxins such as food colouring and all kinds of other additives. And, they offer virtually no nutrition in the form of vitamins and minerals, which are necessary for life. In the long run, that's going to add up to trouble.

If you eat a diet based on good, fresh, healthy food, you are setting the stage for a good, healthy body. You will, in the long run, look better and feel better, and you'll be less likely to suffer from conditions such as cancer, digestive disorders, poor skin and all kinds of other problems. Best of all, fresh foods like fruit and vegetables contain antioxidants, which slow down the process of ageing, so you'll look younger too.

Let's banish one myth here and now. Good food is not dull. In the past, healthy food was considered to be cranky and bland. Not any more. Healthy food is delicious. It tastes far better than prepackaged, processed foods. Good food, that is, food that's good for you, is naturally colourful, full of nutrients and very flavourful. Think of a thick slice of warm wholegrain bread with a little organic butter melted on it. Then picture a thin piece of white toast with margarine. What sounds more delicious: a warm pitta stuffed with marinated chicken breasts, avocado, plump ripe tomatoes and a light yoghurt sauce, or a greasy hamburger? We pop vitamin tablets in some misguided hope that it will make up for poor eating habits. What strange logic: why not eat delicious, nutritious food?

There are many ways to eat well, and to protect your health. This chapter shows you how food can be glorious.

THE NUTS AND BOLTS OF NUTRITION

For literally thousands of years, we have known that food is important for our bodies to function, but it wasn't until this century that we realized why. Nutritional medicine – that is, using nutrition to prevent illness and become healthier – is a fairly new science, and every day we are learning more and more about how food and all its elements work in our bodies.

There are some basic terms that you need to know in order to understand how food is processed in our bodies, and what it does when it gets there. There are two main types of nutrient: macronutrients (the big things that make up the bulk of our food), and micronutrients (tiny quantities of things that are essential for good health).

There are three main macronutrients: fat, carbohydrates and protein. Sometimes nutritionists include water and fibre in this group. Macronutrients provide the body with energy. The body needs micronutrients (vitamins, minerals and other 'trace' substances) in tiny amounts in order to release the energy contained in the macronutrients.

Paula Tilbrook
❀ *Always have loads of fresh fruit and veg at mealtimes – it's amazing how much you can eat of the correct foods without putting on weight. This also will fill you up and give you plenty of nutrients as well as fibre*

FATS

Fats have been given a pretty bad press over the past few years, and if you believed everything you read, you'd think we could do without them. But fats are as important in our diets as any of the other macronutnients, and we could not survive without a certain amount.

Fats are an important source of energy and ensure the smooth functioning of the body, in particular the nervous system. They contain the vitamins A and D and are found in meat, fish, dairy produce and vegetable oils. Fats are stored in special cells that tend to form pads of tissue under the skin and around certain organs and joints. Stored fat serves as a fuel reserve for our body's metabolism, it protects our bodies from shocks and jolts and provides insulation.

There are two kinds of fat. Hard fats, which are solid at room temperature, usually come from an animal source such as fatty meat and dairy food and are referred to as 'saturated fats'.

Oils are liquid at room temperature, and usually come from a plant source. Seeds, nuts and fish oils fall into this category and are referred to as 'unsaturated'.

There are two kinds of unsaturated fats:
- Monounsaturates, like olive oil.
- Polyunsaturates, like corn oil, sunflower oil and peanut (groundnut) oil.

How much do you need? The general opinion is that we need to eat less of all types of fat (good and bad), and change the balance between them. Most people in the West take about 40 per cent of their diet as fat and in Britain it is recommended that fat should provide no more than 35 per cent of our calorie intake. In countries such as Sweden and Canada, even lower proportions have been recommended. If you are a woman of average height and weight, you should probably have no more than about 50 to 80 grams a day.
The good, healthy fats are essential for our bodies to function. They affect the way the brain and nervous system work, and they are also crucial for the immune system, our hormones, our hearts and our skin. The first sign of their deficiency is a dry skin, dry eyes and a greater thirst. Polyunsaturated oils provide two essential fats, known as Omega 6 and Omega 3. Omega 6 is found in sesame seeds, sunflower seeds, evening primrose and borage. Omega 3 is found in pumpkin seeds, linseed, flaxseed and fish oils. You don't need much (only about 2 to 4 tablespoons a day), but they are absolutely crucial for good health.

CARBOHYDRATES

Once again, there are two main groups of carbohydrates – starches and sugars – and one is definitely better for you than the other. Starches, or complex carbohydrates, are turned into sugar by the body. These carbohydrates are found in grains such as wheat, and potatoes and carrots, among other things. Sugars are found in many plants, but table sugar, for example, comes from sugarcane or sugar beet.

Sugars Even if you are pretty sure that your diet is low in sugar, it's important to note that it is often added to food and drink, including soups, tinned fruit and vegetables, baked beans and some meat products. We tend to eat about 25 per cent of our diet as sugar, which is much

too high. Sugars provide calories and usually no other nutrients, and they damage the teeth. Watch out for names like sucrose, glucose and fructose on labels – they all mean the same thing: sugar!

Starches Starches, or complex carbohydrates, are found principally in plant foods, and they are much healthier than sugars. Starch-rich foods, such as wholegrain bread, wholegrain flours, pasta, beans and potatoes are digested slowly by the body, and the sugar is released much more gradually. These foods are also a good source of protein and vitamins and minerals, as well as fibre.
Complex carbohydrates protect your body's muscle stores and let your body use its fat as energy. They should be your main source of energy. When you eat a diet that is high in complex carbohydrates and low in fat, your blood sugar remains stable, which means that your appetite is under control and you will feel more stable emotionally. You should also suffer less from fatigue.

How much do you need? In the West, the starch carbohydrates we eat normally take the form of pasta, bread, flour and potatoes. At the moment, carbohydrates make up about 45 per cent of our diet. Of this, half comes from sugars and the rest from complex carbohydrates. We should be aiming to have about 35 to 70 per cent of our daily calorie intake in the form of complex carbohydrates, avoiding sugars as much as possible.

PROTEIN

Proteins are found in all of our cells, and we need them both to create new cells in our bodies, and to help them work properly. Proteins are made up of amino acids, as well as many hormones, enzymes and other agents involved in metabolism. If you don't get enough protein in your diet, then tissue growth and repair cannot take place, and protein-rich tissue, such as muscle, breaks down. In the West we tend to eat too much protein, and when we take in too much our livers and kidneys are put under a great deal of pressure, and we are more susceptible to certain cancers.

Protein is a critically important part of the diet, mainly because of the amino acids it contains. It's found in foods like pulses, grains, nuts, many vegetables and, most importantly, animal products. Only animal products contain complete protein. That's why it's important to ensure that you get enough protein when you are on a vegetarian or vegan diet. Grains and pulses combine to make a complete protein, as do pulses and nuts.

How much do you need? You need about 60g (2 oz) of protein per day for an average adult. Generally, it's best to eat as much protein as you can from vegetable sources, such as tofu, potatoes, rice and soya, which are lower in saturated fats and more easily digested.

SODIUM

Sodium, an ingredient of salt (sodium chloride), is an essential part of the human diet, helping to regulate body fluids and blood pressure as well as nerve and muscle function and the absorption of other nutrients by the body. Unfortunately, it can be harmful if taken in excess, causing high blood pressure which can lead to heart disease and kidney failure. In the UK, the average daily adult consumption of salt is around nine grams, well over the recommended six grams. Try to cut down on the amount of salt you use when cooking or eliminate it altogether and use herbs, pepper, garlic or lemon for extra flavouring instead. Check the labels of the prepared foods you buy and avoid or cut down on those with high sodium levels, such as bacon, crisps, some breakfast cereals, stock cubes and tinned soups and beans. Be aware that sodium may come from soya, miso or tamari as well as salt. Low salt alternatives are available but you should avoid these if you are diabetic or have kidney disease. Salt can be very dangerous for babies. Don't be tempted to add it to their food.

FIBRE

Dietary fibre, also known as bulk or roughage, is an essential element in the diet even though it provides no nutrients. Fibre is all the indigestible parts of plants. When we chew fibre, it stimulates saliva and it also slows down the passage of food, which means that there is more time for nutrients to be absorbed. It also helps to mop up toxins and fats as it travels through and out of the body. Eating lots of fibre can help to prevent some forms of cancer.

Fruit, vegetables, wholegrain breads, and products made from nuts and pulses are all sources of fibre. In fact, practically all foods of plant origin are useful sources of dietary fibre. The richest sources of fibre are wholemeal bread and flour, peas, beans, dried fruit and nuts.

Fibrous foods help you to feel full for longer and hence reduce the appetite, as well as having other health benefits. For example, they help to control blood sugar levels, since they allow sugar to be released from food more slowly. If you have a good, healthy diet with at least five portions of vegetables and fruit a day, as well as whole grains, you will be getting enough fibre.

VITAMINS AND MINERALS

Vitamins are compounds needed by the body in small quantities to enable growth, development and function. They work with enzymes and other compounds in the body to help produce energy, build tissues, remove waste, and ensure that each system works effectively and efficiently.

Minerals are metals and other inorganic compounds, which work in much the same way as vitamins, promoting body processes, and

Alyson Spiro
✿ *Try to avoid buying packet food. Buy fresh, wholesome food and prepare it at home. It doesn't take that much longer, it is more satisfying and nutritional and it tastes so much better.*
✿ *Listen to your body and go with what it wants. I am a 'grazer'. I just eat little snacks often, and rarely have a big meal. I have more constant energy levels with this way of eating and I do not crave the wrong things or end up bingeing.*

Vitamin	Sources	Function	Therapeutic qualities	Caution
A	Dark green and yellow fruit and vegetables	Needed for strong bones, good vision and healthy skin	Boosts immunity, has anti-cancer effects, fights skin disorders and may reverse ageing of the skin; improves vision; speeds healing; anti-oxidant	Vitamin A is toxic in excess and may cause birth defects if taken during pregnancy
B1 (Thiamine)	All plant and animal foods, including wholegrain products, brown rice, seafood and beans	Converts blood sugar into energy; promotes growth and is a nervous tonic	Protects against damage caused by alcohol, treats anaemia, may help to improve IQ and memory, may help to control diabetes	In very high doses, vitamin B1 can be toxic
B2 (Riboflavin)	Meat, milk and dairy produce, green leafy vegetables, fruit, bread, cereals	Essential for the production of energy, and is an antioxidant	Protects against cancer, protects against anaemia, boosts athletic performance	May be toxic in very high doses
B3 (Niacin)	Meats, fish and poultry	Essential for sex hormones, increases energy, aids nervous system, helps digestion	Lowers cholesterol, may relieve migraine headaches and arthritis, reduces high blood pressure	Toxic in high doses
B5 (Pantothenic Acid)	Organ meats, fish, eggs, wholegrain cereals	Aids in healing wounds, fights infection, strengthens immune system, builds cells	Boosts energy and athletic prowess, lowers cholesterol levels, prevents and treats arthritis, speeds the healing of wounds, detoxifies alcohol, stimulates immunity, retards the ageing process	None
B6 (Pyridoxine)	Meats, wholegrains and yeast	Required for the functioning of more than 60 enzymes, aids the nervous system and the production of cells crucial for a healthy immune system	Boosts immunity, protects against cancer, relieves the symptoms of PMS (pre-menstrual syndrome) and infertility, may prevent some skin diseases, prevents against nervous disorders	Do not exceed 50 mg per day
B12 (Cyanocolbalamin)	Fish, dairy produce, organic meats, eggs	Forms and regenerates red blood cells, increases energy, improves concentration, maintains nervous system.	Energizes the body, protects against some cancers, protects against toxins and allergens	Toxic in high doses
Folic Acid	Fresh leaf green vegetables, yeasts and liver	For red blood cell formation in bone marrow, crucial to normal functioning of nervous system and normal production of genetic material	Protects against cancer, prevents birth defects, may help in the treatment of atherosclerosis	Toxic in large doses

Vitamin	Sources	Function	Therapeutic qualities	Caution
C	Fresh fruit and vegetables, potatoes, leafy herbs and berries	Vital for healthy skin, bones, muscles, healing and protection from viruses, toxins, drugs; an effective antioxidant	Fights cancer, boosts immune system, lowers cholesterol, speeds healing of wounds, helps maintain good vision, may help to overcome male infertility, counteracts asthma	May cause kidney stones, gout, diarrhoea and cramps in excess
D	Milk produce, eggs, fatty fish, fish oil Synthesized in the skin from sunlight	Vital for normal calcium formation and growth, and health of bone and teeth. Increases absorption of calcium from diet	Protects against cancer, beneficial in the treatment of cancer, enhances immunity and used in the treatment of some skin disorders. Protects against osteoporosis	Toxic in high doses
E	Nuts, seeds, eggs, milk, wholegrains, unrefined oils, leafy vegetables, avocados, and soya	Essential for absorption of iron, metabolism of essential fatty acids; protects the circulatory system and cells, slows the ageing process, increases fertility and protects against foetal abnormalities	Protects against neurological disorders, boosts the immune system, is antioxidant, protects against cancer, heart and breast diseases, reduces the symptoms of PMS (pre-menstrual syndrome), fights skin problems, reduces muscular cramps, prevents miscarriage,	Toxic in very high doses, and may elevate blood pressure
K	Green vegetables, milk products, molasses, apricots, wholegrains, cod liver oil Synthesized in the intestines	Produces blood clotting factors	May help in the treatment of cancer, protects against osteoporosis	Toxic in very high doses

MINERALS

Mineral	Sources	Functions	Therapeutic uses	Cautions
Boron	Pears, prunes, pulses, raisins, tomatoes, apples	Helps to maintain mineral levels and hormones needed for bone health. May help to reduce calcium loss in post menopausal women. Prevents osteoporosis. Builds muscle	Arthritis, osteoporosis, menopause symptoms, muscle building, external treatment of fungal and bacterial infections	Toxic above about 100 mg
Calcium	Milk, cheese and dairy produce, leafy green vegetables, salmon, nuts, root vegetables, broccoli and tofu	Necessary for action of some hormones and of muscles, necessary for blood pressure regulation and clotting; strong bones and teeth; helps metabolize iron	Growing pains, menstrual cramps, hypoglycaemia, muscle cramps, osteoporosis, allergies, high blood pressure, migraine, heart problems, insommia	Doses over 2,000 mg per day may cause hyperglycaemia

Mineral	Sources	Functions	Therapeutic uses	Cautions
Chromium	Liver, wholegrain cereals, meat and cheese, brewer's yeast, molasses, mushrooms, and egg yolk	Chromium works in the body to stimulate insulin activity, stabilize blood sugar levels; regulate appetite	High cholesterol levels, hypoglycaemia, diabetes, heart disease, depression/ anxiety, PMS-related symptoms	Some people experience troubled dreams when taking chromium supplements
Cobalt	Fresh leafy green vegetables, meat, liver, milk, oysters and clams	Works with vitamin B12 in: the production of red blood cells; the health of the nervous system	Only used as a part of B12 to prevent pernicious anaemia, helps in the production of red blood cells; nervous system problems	In excess cobalt or its compounds can cause nausea, damage to the heart, kidneys, and nerves, and even death
Copper	Avocados, animal livers, molasses, whole grains, shellfish, nuts, fruit, oysters, kidneys and legumes	Helps iron absorption; Necessary for: production of adrenal hormones; to maintain blood vessels and connective tissues; for the production of energy; antioxidant, maintains nerve fibres; essential for utilization of vitamin C	Anaemia, rheumatism and arthritis, some cancers, energy problems	Excess intake can cause vomiting, diarrhoea, muscular pain, depression, irritability, nervousness and dementia, but toxicity is low and very rare
Fluorine	Seafood, animal meat, black tea	Protects against dental cavities; may help to prevent heart disease	Tooth decay, weak bones, osteoporosis	10 to 80 mg is considered to be a toxic dose, which can cause serious tooth and bone problems. Slightly lower doses may cause energy problems
Iodine	Fish and seafood, pineapple, raisins, seaweed, dairy produce	Prevents goitre; produces hormones from thyroid gland, promotes healthy hair, skin, nails, teeth; burns excess fat	Cuts and wounds (as an antiseptic, used externally), goitre, fibrocystic breast disease, thyroid problems	Iodine is toxic in high doses and may aggravate or cause acne. Large doses may interfere with hormone activity
Iron	Liver, kidneys, raw clams, cocoa powder, dark chocolate, shellfish, pulses, broccoli, nuts, egg yolks, red meat, beans and molasses	Necessary for: production of haemoglobin and certain enzymes, immune activity; protects against some free radicals	Anaemia, hearing loss, period pain, restless leg syndrome, growth problems, poor resistance to infection, fatigue	Toxicity is rare, but excess iron can cause constipation
Magnesium	Brown rice, soya beans, nuts, brewer's yeast, whole grains, bitter chocolate and legumes	Repairs and maintains body cells; required for hormonal activity; required for most body processes, including energy production; antidiabetic; required for contraction and relaxation of muscles, including heart; necessary for bone development	Kidney stones, asthma, osteoporosis, depression and anxiety, energy problems, fibromyalgia, glaucoma, diabetes, PMS, period pains, hypoglycaemia, insomnia, migraine, gum disease, eclampsia, hearing loss, high blood pressure, prostate problems, high cholesterol	Magnesium is toxic to people with renal problems or atrioventricular blocks

Mineral	Sources	Functions	Therapeutic uses	Cautions
Manganese	Cereals, tea, green leaf vegetables, wholemeal bread, pulses, liver, root vegetables, and nuts	Necessary for the functioning of the brain; used in the treatment of some nervous disorders; necessary for normal bone structure; important in the formation of thyroxin, in the thyroid gland	Epilepsy, Alzheimer's and schizophrenia, anaemia, diabetes, heart disease, atherosclerosis, arthritis	None
Molybdenum	Buckwheat, canned beans, wheat germ, liver, pulses, whole grains, offal and eggs	Aids metabolism of fats and carbohydrates; protects against cancer; prevents anaemia and impotence; protects against dental cavities	Anaemia, impotence	Molybdenum is toxic in doses higher than 10-15 mg, which causes goutlike symptoms
Phosphorus	Meat, fish, yeast, whole grains, cheese, soya products, nuts	Forms bones, teeth and cell membranes; produces energy; burns sugar for energy; increases endurance	Conditions listed above that are caused or exacerbated by a disease-related phosphorous deficiency	Toxic
Potassium	Avocados, leafy green vegetables, bananas, dried fruits, fruit and vegetable juices, soya flour, potatoes, nuts and molasses	Necessary for transportation of carbon dioxide by red blood cells; required for water balance and protein synthesis	None	In excess may cause muscular weakness and mental apathy, eventually stopping the heart. It may also cause ulceration of the small intestine
Selenium	Wheat germ, bran, tuna fish, onions, tomatoes, broccoli and wholemeal bread	Antioxidant necessary for DNA repair; required by the immune system; prevents many cancers; improves liver function; maintains healthy eyes and eyesight; maintains healthy skin and hair; protects against heart and circulatory diseases; may impede the ageing process; can detoxify alcohol, many drugs, smoke and some fats; increases male potency and sex drive	Dandruff, arthritis, cancers, AIDS, asthma, sperm motility, thyroid function, kidney problems, muscular dystrophy, acne, hepatitis, and epilepsy	Toxic in small doses
Zinc	Offal, meat, mushrooms, seeds, nuts, oysters, eggs, wholegrain products and brewer's yeast	Required for male fertility, hormones, immunity, growth, energy metabolism, haemoglobin; detoxifies alcohol; prevents cancer; may help prevent degenerative effects of ageing including blindness; antioxidant	Male infertility, acne, anorexia, mouth ulcers, viral infections, herpes, sickle cell anaemia, tinnitus, thyroid function, immune problems, arthritis, ulcers, growth problems, cancer, allergies, alcoholism	Zinc is thought to be non-toxic, although very high doses (above 150 mg per day) may cause some nausea, vomiting and diarrhoea

providing much of the structure for teeth and bones. Minerals are classified in two groups – proper or major minerals, needed in quantities of over 100 mg per day, and minor minerals, or trace elements, which are required by the body in quantities of less than 100 mg per day.

There are some 15 vitamins and 18 minerals that have been isolated as being essential for normal body functions. These nutrients work together to keep the body functioning at optimum level. When one or more is in short supply, the body cannot function properly and health problems occur.

The vitamins we need are divided into two categories: water-soluble vitamins (the B vitamins and vitamin C) and fat-soluble vitamins (A, D, E, and K). The water-soluble vitamins are absorbed by the intestine and carried to the tissues where they will be put into use. Because water-soluble vitamins are not stored in the body, they must be taken daily to prevent deficiency.

Fat-soluble vitamins have specialized functions. They are absorbed by the intestine and the lymphatic system carries them to the different parts of the body. The body can store larger amounts of fat-soluble vitamins than of water-soluble vitamins, so excessive intake of fat-soluble vitamins, particularly vitamins A and D, can lead to toxic levels in the body.

Pages 22–25 show the most common vitamins and minerals found in foods and in supplements. The foods with the highest content of each nutrient are listed under 'sources'. The function column explains why we need each nutrient. Therapeutic qualities refers to the conditions and symptoms that the vitamin or mineral can alleviate or treat, when eaten as part of a healthy diet, or when supplemented. Cautions are really only relevant if you plan to take supplements, but it's important to note what to expect when you do get too much, or which health conditions preclude too much of a particular nutrient.

ANTIOXIDANTS

Nutrients called antioxidants – which are contained in fruit, nuts and most vegetables, are the body's defence against what scientists call

OTHER SUPPLEMENTS

AMINO ACIDS

Amino acids are compounds that make up the 'building blocks' of protein. If we eat enough different types of protein we should be getting enough in our diet. Health problems can occur when we get all of our proteins from, say, animal sources, rather than a mix of plant and animal sources. Amino acids are necessary to make all the elements in the body, including hair, skin, bone, tissues, antibodies, hormones, enzymes and blood. They also help to regulate energy and perform other functions. Amino acids can be taken as supplements for various health conditions, but you should never consider taking one without the advice of a registered practitioner.

ROYAL JELLY

Royal jelly has been used for centuries for its health-giving and rejuvenating properties, and it is rich in vitamins, amino acids and minerals. It is also the prime source of fatty acid, which is said to increase alertness and act as a natural tranquillizer (when necessary). Royal jelly is secreted in the salivary glands of the worker bees to feed and stimulate the growth and development of the queen bee. Humans use it for a variety of reasons, including its ability to prevent yeast from building up (very useful in the treatment of thrush), and in the treatment of allergies, some cancers, fatigue, low immunity and skin problems. Royal Jelly is

safe to take as a supplement, but avoid it if you have an allergy to bee stings.

ACIDOPHILUS

There are certain types of bacteria that are considered healthy. They work to ensure that the bacteria in our bodies are balanced. After a course of antibiotics, for example, good bacteria as well as unhealthy bacteria may have been killed off, and you become more susceptible to tummy bugs, viruses and yeast infections, such as thrush, which the healthy bacteria would normally control. Acidophilus and other healthy bacteria, such as bifidus, help to keep the intestines clean, help us to absorb the nutrients from our food, prevent constipation and flatulence, help in the treatment of acne and other skin problems, and help to keep yeast infections at bay. Acidophilus is found in live yoghurt, and if you take a couple of spoonfuls every day, it will contribute to good bowel health, among other things. There are also supplements available and drinks, such as Yakult, which contain acidophilus. If you suffer from digestive complaints or thrush, it's a good idea to include these in your diet on a daily basis, particularly after you have taken antibiotics.

CO-ENZYME Q10

Co-enzyme Q10 is a vitamin-like substance found in all cells of the body. Studies show that it enhances our immunity, may help to prevent heart problems, helps to slow down the process of ageing, boosts energy levels and is necessary for our brains and nervous systems to function properly. Many people use it to boost their memories. It's a safe supplement to take, but you can get it from spinach, cold water fish, such as tuna, and organ meats. If these foods don't feature regularly in your diet, you might want to consider supplementing.

GARLIC
Garlic is a herb and a member of the onion family. It can be eaten fresh, or taken as a supplement for some pretty amazing health benefits. We know, for example, that garlic helps to cleanse the blood and keep healthy bacteria active in the gut. It also helps to bring down a fever, tone the heart (preventing all kinds of heart problems), treat infections (viral and bacterial), reduce blood pressure, boost the immune system and prevent the effects of ageing. It may also help to prevent some cancers. If you aren't including garlic in your diet, now's the time to do so. If you can't bear the taste, odourless capsules are available.

ECHINACEA
Echinacea is a versatile herb that can be taken internally and applied externally to fight bacterial and viral infections, lower fever and calm allergic reactions. It is one of the most popular immune stimulants, and studies show that it is extremely effective in promoting healing, and

fighting such infectious conditions as flu, candidiasis, colds and herpes. Echinacea is best taken in small, frequent doses, especially during the flu season, or if you are feeling run down. If used in the long-term, take for only six days out of seven, or three weeks out of four, for best effect.

FISH OILS
Fish oils are a great source of essential fatty acids (EFAs), and they may help to prevent cancer (especially breast cancer) and arthritis, protect against heart disease and high blood pressure, and treat skin disorders, such as psoriasis. If you eat plenty of oily fish, such as tuna, mackerel, herring and salmon, you are probably getting enough. If you don't, this is one supplement worth taking.

EVENING PRIMROSE
Evening primrose oil is another source of EFAs, especially Omega 6, and it has a whole host of healing benefits. For one thing, it is now proven to reduce the symptoms of PMS when taken regularly, long-term. It is also terrific for treating skin conditions such as eczema and psoriasis. It discourages dry skin, helps to treat asthma, can help your liver to regenerate (very useful if you've had a period of drinking a bit too much), and can help to stimulate the body to convert fat into energy (in other words, lose weight!) If you suffer from any of the above conditions, take 300 mg daily. Safflower oil is also rich in Omega 6.

Paul Loughran
✿ *My weight started to increase with all the large breakfasts and lunches we get on location, plus I would go home at night and eat a big evening meal. I cut out the evening meal and lost the extra weight. It is best to fuel your body during the day, when you need the energy and can use it, not when you are just about to go to bed and it will turn to fat.*

free radicals, molecules which have become unstable and which oxidize neighbouring molecules, causing all types of cellular damage in the body. Free radicals are implicated in cancer, heart disease, and even ageing itself – so much so that many experts believe the ageing process is actually produced by the constant, tiny degenerative effects caused by free radicals as they oxidize various cells over time. The most powerful antioxidants are Vitamins E and C, as well as Vitamin A and its precursor betacarotene, and the minerals selenium and zinc. Ensure you get these nutrients in your diet, and you can set yourself up for a future of good health.

THE FOOD PYRAMID
Now that we have a good understanding of the important parts of our diet, it's time to put that information into practice. Looking down the long list of essential nutrients, you could be forgiven for thinking that you'll never manage to squeeze them all into your diet. The good news is that with a healthy diet, based on a system called the food pyramid, you should get almost all of what you need. Shortfalls can be addressed by taking a good multi-vitamin and mineral tablet, and some of the extra supplements that you think seem appropriate for your general health and well being.

So what is the food pyramid? To reflect research findings on nutrition, the daily diet recommendations were changed in 1992 from the square of the four food groups to a food pyramid, with foods that should be eaten more often at the base, and those less frequently consumed at the top. The emphasis is on eating less of the groups' meat and meat substitutes, dairy products and oils and fats, and more of breads and cereals, and fruit and vegetables. Some scientists feel that these recommendations do not go far enough and are pressing for the near elimination of meat and fats from the Western diet.

This pyramid is a practical tool to help you make food choices that are consistent with the dietary guidelines recommended by the government. It encourages you to eat a variety of different foods every day to make sure you get all the nutrients you need. To make the most of the pyramid, you need to know what constitutes a serving:

FOOD GROUP	SERVING SIZE
Bread	1 slice bread, ½ bagel or muffin, 25 g (1 oz) ready-to-eat cereal, ½ cup porridge, rice or pasta, or 5-6 crackers or oatcakes
Vegetables	1 cup raw, leafy vegetables, ½ cup cooked or chopped raw vegetables or 180 ml (6 oz) vegetable juice
Fruit	1 medium piece of fruit, ½ cup mixed fruit or 180 ml (6oz) fruit juice
Milk	180 ml (6oz) milk or yoghurt, 40 g (1½ oz) cheese
Meat	50-75 g (2-3oz) cooked lean meat, poultry or fish (about the size of a deck of playing cards)

Other foods that count as a serving from the second row include ½ cup cooked beans, 1 egg, 2 tablespoons peanut butter or ⅓ cup nuts. If you don't have a set of cups, use a measuring jug. One cup equals 250 ml or, if you use Imperial measurements, a scant nine fluid ounces.

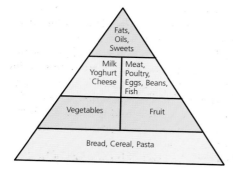

WHAT SHOULD WE EAT AND WHEN?

Most of us have been brought up to believe that we should eat three good, nutritious meals every day, starting with a healthy breakfast. Increasingly, however, we are learning that it's much healthier to eat when we are hungry, rather than filling up on meals that we may not need. Today, many of us lead fairly sedentary lifestyles, and we just don't need the amount of food that we once did.

Using the food pyramid as a guide, plan your meals in advance so that you always have plenty of fresh fruit and vegetables available for when you are hungry. Eating well does not mean starving yourself. Listen to your body. If you are hungry six times a day, eat six small meals. If you need a snack mid-afternoon or in the evening, choose something satisfying from the food pyramid. The important thing to remember is that you should eat when you are hungry, focusing on the healthy options. If your routine doesn't fit in with that of your family, choose something small and light for table-time and concentrate on eating when your body tells you to.

FOOD ALLERGIES AND INTOLERANCE

Food allergies and intolerances are escalating, and recently, 'intolerances', which are a milder form of allergy, have been recognized as a fundamental cause of many common ailments, including eczema, dermatitis and asthma, all of which have increased dramatically over recent years. The most common symptoms of intolerances are migraine, fatigue, depression, anxiety, hyperactivity in children, mouth ulcers, aching muscles, water retention, wind, joint pain, rheumatoid arthritis, nausea, vomiting, gastric ulcers, Crohn's disease, abdominal bloating, irritable bowel syndrome and constipation. Feel like you are a likely candidate? Read on.

You may find that when you are run down – say after suffering from a series of colds, stressful circumstances, or a bout of flu – you are more susceptible to intolerances and allergies. Perfumes or make-up that are normally used may cause you to break out in a rash, or your pet may suddenly make you sneeze – this means that your immune system, which is under strain or depleted, has decided to respond to 'normal' things in an 'abnormal' way. In many cases, allergies or intolerances can be temporary, and indeed, long-term sufferers of hay fever, asthma, eczema and allergies to common foods find that taking steps to boost their immune systems, and live healthier lifestyles, cause 'allergies' to disappear altogether.

Food allergies and intolerances are particularly difficult to pinpoint as a cause of illness, and many of us are intolerant without knowing it. If you crave certain foods, and these foods form a major part of your daily diet, you may well be intolerant. People who have had difficulty shifting weight, or who suffer from overwhelming fatigue, sleep disturbances, dry skin or food cravings often experience a complete alleviation of symptoms when they remove suspect foods (often foods that are craved or overeaten) from their daily diets. In most cases, excess weight, bloating and fatigue disappear, and they feel much healthier overall. This doesn't mean that suspect foods need to be avoided for ever – they should be eaten as 'treats', rather than used as staples of the diet, and they should be avoided when you are feeling run-down, tired, bloated or even depressed.

What can you do? Food allergies and intolerances are often difficult to assess, and your doctor can run a series of tests if you suspect that you are intolerant or even just sensitive to some foods. Anyone who suffers from the common ailments listed above should consider the possibility of food being the root cause, and take steps to eliminate suspect elements of the diet. You can carry out an informal test at home if you are concerned about a certain food. It is important to maintain a balanced diet, so strict elimination or exclusion diets should only be carried out

Steve Magan
✿ *Eat pasta. So many people think it is an enemy, but carbohydrate is not fattening, so long as you eat it with a healthy tomato-based sauce and don't laden it with cream sauces and Parmesan cheese.*
✿ *I never bother with fancy, low fat margarines, which I feel are laden with preservatives and additives. I would much rather have normal butter, but just a bit of it. I think it is better for me.*

under reputable professional supervision. Keep a food diary throughout a period of exclusion so that you can look back at your patterns of eating and symptoms. Introduce foods in small quantities, one at a time, to see if you get any kind of a reaction before having normal helpings again.

ENJOY!
Food can be absolutely sensuous. When you eat what you want, when you are hungry (bearing in mind, of course, that three chocolate bars do not constitute the healthiest of diets), you are much more likely to be satisfied than you would be if you ate a meal you didn't particularly fancy.

A recent study showed that people who cook their own meals often need to eat less, primarily because their senses have been sated. Half of eating is the pleasure of smelling and tasting it. When our brains receive signals that something tasty is in the oven, we begin to salivate. Just a few tastes are often enough to send a message to our appetite control centre that the mission has been accomplished. We no longer feel hungry.

Bear this in mind when you are considering your meals. Although it is undoubtedly easier to throw a pre-cooked meal into the oven, you are doing little to satisfy the sensory part of the eating process. Consider this: what sounds more appealing? A frozen lasagne in a foil tin, or a steaming dish of pasta with fresh vegetable sauce, basil, mozzarella cheese and pine nuts? We have become so accustomed to substituting convenience for taste that the first option may well sound easier. The fact is that the second option can be cooked inside 15 minutes. It is also more nutritious, satisfying and, most importantly, delicious.

Get into the habit of buying lots of fresh

vegetables to have on hand for easy-to-prepare meals. Take chicken breasts or lean meats out of the freezer the night before, throw them in a plastic container with a bit of honey, olive oil, a few squirts of lemon juice and some salt and pepper, and leave them in a cool place, ready to cook the next day. Fifteen to 20 minutes in the oven – as long as it takes to cook any ready-prepared meal – will produce the perfect, moist chicken breast. Chop it up and stir fry in a little olive oil for even faster results. Cook extra for lunch or dinner the next day.

Keep fresh tomatoes in a glass bowl on a sunny window sill to ensure that they are juicy and flavoursome. Chop up two or three large tomatoes, heat a little olive oil in a pan and fry them lightly until the juice just runs. Throw in a little fresh basil, some sea salt and pepper and serve with a sprinkling of pine nuts and a few cubes of low-fat mozzarella cheese.

If you feel a craving for something sweet, choose the most delicious piece of chocolate cake you can find – something you'll really enjoy – and eat it slowly, savouring every morsel. Or buy a ripe, succulent mango and eat it with a bowl of Greek yoghurt and honey. Eat things that inspire you. Plan meals that make your mouth water. You'll find you need to eat a lot less of something completely delicious than you would of something simply placed in front of you.

VEGETARIANS AND VEGANS

Increasingly more people are turning to an exclusively or a predominantly vegetarian diet. In the UK there are an estimated 5 million vegetarians and millions more who have stopped eating red meat.

Despite popular criticism, a vegetarian diet is a perfectly healthy diet so long as adequate nutrients, including protein (see page 20), are eaten. As long as your diet is not restricted, it is fairly easy to eat healthily. The stumbling block for many vegetarians is protein intake. A vegetarian diet should contain a variety of foods, such as cereals, beans, nuts, pulses and vegetables, to ensure a good balance of proteins and other nutrients. Cereals, beans, pulses and nuts should predominate in the diet, particularly

if fewer dairy products are consumed. These foods are rich in protein and will ensure that adequate quantities are available for the processes of the body, including the rebuilding of the body's tissues. Lack of iron can also be a problem, particularly for teenagers. Increased amounts of beans, pulses, nuts, dried fruit or wholegrain cereals should help to overcome this problem, and fresh fruit and vegetables will provide the vitamin C necessary for the iron to be absorbed.

A HEALTHY VEGETARIAN DIET

Ensure that your diet includes something from each of the following groups:

- **Complex carbohydrates**
  Pasta, bread, rice, potatoes, cereals, wholegrains
- **Fruit and vegetables**
  Fruit, fruit juice, vegetables, including potatoes
- **Dairy proteins**
  Cheese, milk, yoghurt
- **Animal and vegetable proteins**
  Eggs, nuts, seeds, pulses, tofu, soya products

VEGANS

A vegan diet, which does not include any animal products, contains even more bulk than a vegetarian diet, and it is therefore more difficult to ensure that you get the required nutritional elements, and calories. The most common nutrients lacking in a vegan diet are calcium, vitamin D and vitamin B12. A vegan diet does not provide vitamin B12 in sufficient quantities. B12 is found mainly in animal products, with the exception of miso, tempeh, brewer's yeast and soya milks that have been fortified. The latter foods cannot be eaten in large enough quantities to provide the required daily intake, so it is recommended that all vegans take a vitamin B12 supplement.

Calcium is found in a variety of non-dairy foods, but it is important to ensure that these foods are eaten regularly. High-calcium foods include broccoli, soya beans, almonds, tofu, soya milk (or soya yoghurt and cheese), dried fruits and dark green vegetables.

HEALTHY DRINKING

There's nothing better than a glass of wine at the end of a day. Instant relaxation, much less expensive than a trip to your acupuncturist and blissfully delicious. The problem is, you are probably likely to feel guilty. We've all been warned about the problems associated with alcohol, and you have to be a mental maths wizard to be able to tot up units when you are out on the town.

Alcohol is, in reasonable quantities, good for you. As a tool for stress-relief, it's probably not the ideal way to relax every single day, and it can be addictive. But studies show that a moderate intake of alcohol, say a glass a day, is good for your health. If you rarely overindulge, seldom have a hangover but you do sip a soothing glass of wine at the end of the day, chances are you will live longer, and experience a better quality of life. One glass (unit) of alcohol a day helps to relieve stress, to fend off heart disease, and promotes longevity. Eric Rimm, a nutritional epidemiologist at the Harvard University School of Public Health in Boston, says: 'If someone can control alcohol consumption, then a glass of wine, a can of beer or a mixed drink a day can extend his or her life. In fact, death rates for people who savour a drink a day are 16 per cent lower than for men or women who either drink more or nothing at all.' Recently, this research has been disputed, but there are an overwhelming number of studies that suggest that alcohol – like anything else – in moderation is good for long-term health.

THE UNIT SYSTEM

One unit of drink is half a pint of average strength beer (about 4 per cent), or a single of 70 per cent proof spirit, or one glass of wine. One unit contains 8 grams of ethanol (pure alcohol). So someone drinking 80 grams of ethanol (a heavy drinker) a day is taking about five pints of beer, or five double whiskies or a bottle of wine.

The answer is, as with everything else: find a balance. It's much worse for you to binge on wine than it is to have a regular drink or two in the evening. Having said that, a very occasional binge is not going to ruin your health irrevocably either. Have a drink if it makes you feel good, but learn how to stop before that feeling turns sour – or causes a nasty hangover the next day.

There's more to life than alcohol, however, and we need to consider the other things on the drinks menu. What should we be drinking and how much?

WATER

Pure, fresh, filtered water is your number one bet. It's likely to be free of bacteria, pesticides and other nasties, and it will quench your thirst without putting any strain on your body. That means your body will be able to eliminate toxins easily, without having to put in any hard work. The more you drink, the less water you retain (honestly! water is the best diuretic known), and the better your body will function. Aim for eight to ten biggish glasses every day. Try to start your day with a glass of lukewarm water to get your liver going. I always drink at least a litre and a half of mineral water a day – people have commented that the mineral water bottle is my trademark. I find it helps my skin stay clear and healthy too. If you are thirsty then you are already dehydrating – keep hydrated.

FIZZY DRINKS

Big no-no really. Think about what is contained in, for example, a can of cola. Water and chemicals. There is no nutritional value in fizzy drinks. If they are not a 'diet' brand, they will contain about eight to ten tablespoons of sugar (more than you should have in an entire day, really), probably some caffeine and lots of lovely e-numbers. Diet drinks aren't really any better. Most of them contain chemicals that are designed to make you feel full. Great on a diet, you may think, but the fact is that they can cause bloating and may even slow down your body's metabolism, making it harder to lose weight. A recent study in the US

Malandra Burrows
✿ *To lose weight, eat less! Cut out nibbling between meals and if you really are starving eat a piece of fruit to keep going.*

SUPERFOODS!

Superfoods are known as 'functional foods', and they do much more than provide us with energy to live and to grow. Functional foods have therapeutic properties, which means they can work to balance and to heal our bodies. Best of all, these substances are natural, they have no side-effects and they can be as effective as many drugs. By incorporating these natural, easy-to-grow and purchase foods in your daily diet, you can improve your health on all levels, and treat common ailments, such as asthma, eczema, constipation and fatigue. Read on!

APPLES
■ A mild diuretic and laxative, and are therefore useful for the treatment of constipation.
■ Cleanse teeth and encourage gum health.
■ The pectin and vitamin C in apples helps to reduce cholesterol levels
■ May reduce indigestion, and help your body to metabolize protein and fats.
■ Are excellent detoxifiers, and useful in the treatment of diarrhoea and other digestive disorders.
■ Are antiseptic, anti-viral and a great tonic.

AVOCADOS
■ Are rich in vitamins A, B-complex, C and E.
■ Are excellent for circulatory disorders, convalescence, fatigue and stress.
■ Reduce the effects of ageing on the skin.
■ Contain antibacterial and anti-fungal substances.

BANANAS
■ Help the body to eliminate toxins and waste.
■ Are a rich source of vitamin B6.
■ Ripe bananas help to build up natural bacteria in the bowel (called flora) which help fight off infections.
■ Are excellent for lifting spirits and fighting fatigue; useful for convalescence.

BROCCOLI
■ Protects against cancer – particularly cancers of the digestive system.
■ Protects against heart disease and treats joint problems.
■ Is rich in iron, which is useful to treat anaemia and for people suffering from chronic fatigue.

CABBAGE
■ Raw cabbage is a traditional cure for ulcers.
■ Has disinfectant properties for respiratory conditions.
■ Is rich in iron, and protects against stress, infections and heart disease.

CARROTS
■ Are rich in vitamin A (as beta carotene), which aids respiration and treats skin and eye problems.
■ Protect against cancer.
■ Carrot juice is recommended for liver problems.
■ May slow down the ageing process, and prevent heart disease.

CRANBERRIES
■ Treat cystitis and other urinary system infections.
■ Are high in vitamin C and other vitamins and minerals.
■ May prevent kidney stones.

GARLIC
■ Is anti-bacterial, anti-fungal and anti-viral and an anti-oxidant.
■ Protects against cancer.
■ Draws out abscesses.
■ Draws out pain.
■ Is an excellent tonic.
■ Lowers blood pressure and cholesterol levels.
■ Is used in the treatment of asthma.

GRAPES
■ Are cleansing and regenerative.
■ Are excellent for anaemia, fatigue and joint disorders, which may be the result of inadequate elimination.
■ Grapeseed oil is rich in vitamin E.

■ Drink the juice during periods of stress, fatigue and illness of any kind to aid health and prevent respiratory infections.
■ Can be used to treat infant diarrhoea, and to soothe an inflamed bowel.

pointed out that diet soft drinks were one of the main reasons why women found it so difficult to lose weight. They hamper the process, not help it. If you are a caffeine fiend, make yourself a glass of iced tea with lemon. If you can't go a day without a cola, make sure you drink plenty of water in and around it to flush the system. Better still, avoid it completely if you can.

COFFEE AND TEA
Sorry, folks, but coffee and tea are toxic. One of the best-known toxins in both is caffeine. Tea contains about 60 per cent of the caffeine of coffee. Obviously that's the attraction of both tea and coffee. For the record, chocolate contains about the same. Caffeine is not all bad – it stimulates the brain, helping to keep you awake, and it is also a diuretic, which means that it stimulates the flow of urine.

The odd cup of coffee will not hurt you. Moderate intake (say a cup or two a day) is all right, as long as you drink plenty of water in and around it, to help flush out the many toxins it provides. Too much coffee, however, can cause big problems. Irregular heartbeat, confusion, ringing in the ears and stomach upsets are not uncommon for big coffee drinkers, and if it doesn't make it more difficult for you to get to sleep, it will certainly make your sleep less restful. Stick to as few cups a day as you can manage.

Decaffeinated coffee may be lower in caffeine, but it is not any better for you. Indeed, the process of decaffeinating actually increases

■ Treat skin problems, and may encourage metabolism.

HONEY
■ Is antibacterial – used externally and internally.
■ Honey with apple cider vinegar is a perfect tonic and detoxifier.
■ May shift some types of arthritis deposits.
■ Is nutritious, and a natural antihistamine.
■ Offsets respiratory problems.
■ Overcomes fatigue.

LEMONS
■ Are anti-infectious – used to treat viruses, coughs, colds and other respiratory and bacterial infections.
■ Purify the blood
■ Lemon juice can be used to detoxify arthritis and rheumatic patients.
■ Lemon juice can control some bladder and kidney infections.
■ Protect the digestive tract.
■ Are rich in vitamin C, and some B vitamins.
■ Are a skin cleanser (used internally), and regulate digestion.
■ Stimulate the immune system.

NUTS
■ Are excellent for convalescence, and to improve virility.
■ Are extremely nutritious, with protein, vitamin B1 and magnesium, which are vital to the nervous system.

OATS
■ Heal internally.
■ Help promote strong bones and teeth.
■ Lower blood cholesterol levels.
■ Are nervine, which means they address the health of the nervous system.
■ Are nutritious – with vitamin E and B-complex vitamins, calcium, potassium, and magnesium.
■ Soothe intestinal and digestive disorders.
■ Are used to treat depression, chronic fatigue and general debility, are said to have a tranquillizing effect.

OLIVE OIL
■ Has an antioxidant effect, which can slow down the ageing process and prevent degenerative diseases.
■ Is excellent for skin conditions – taken internally, or used externally.
■ May help to expel

gallstones.
■ Is recommended for liver problems.
■ Reduces cholesterol levels, and protects against heart disease.

ONIONS
■ Are diuretic and have antibiotic activity.
■ Lower blood sugar levels.
■ Prevent blood cholesterol.
■ Reduce tendency for blood to clot.
■ Are used to treat bronchitis, anaemia, asthma and ageing, arthritis, gout and colic.

ORANGES
■ Boost immunity.
■ Are excellent for convalescence, and may help to reduce the spread of some cancers.
■ Are rich in vitamin C, vitamin A and bioflavonoids.
■ Strengthen the walls of the capillaries.
■ Are used to treat respiratory conditions, colds, flu and coughs.

RICE
■ Aids circulation.
■ Lowers blood pressure.
■ Soothes and cleanses the digestive tract.
■ Is useful for the

treatment of fatigue and stress.

STRAWBERRIES
■ Cleanse and regenerate.
■ Are high in iron, which makes them good for anaemia and fatigue.
■ Lower high blood pressure.
■ May help to eliminate kidney stones.
■ Are restorative, and stimulate the body and heart.
■ May ease skin problems.

YOGHURT
■ Eases fatigue.
■ Live yoghurt is an excellent antiseptic and anti-fungal agent and can be applied directly to the vagina for thrush, and any itching caused by urinary infections.
■ Natural 'live' yoghurt will help to restore the body's natural bacteria (flora), which aid digestion, regulate excretion, and fights infection.

the chemical content, making it a stronger toxin.

Tea is a slightly different story. Tea does have some healthy properties, and as long as you don't drink it too strong, should be lower in caffeine than coffee. Black tea contains tannins, which are believed to help prevent some forms of heart disease. Tea also contains a little natural fluoride, which is good for your teeth. Green tea is believed to improve resistance to stomach and skin cancers, and stimulates the immune system. Once again, however, everything in moderation. Too much tea is as bad for you as too much coffee. If you drink lots of tea, increase your intake of water.

HERBAL TEAS AND TISANES
These are a much healthier option. Not only do

they have no toxins in them, but they also have plenty of healthy properties. They cleanse and strengthen the body, and have a wide range of therapeutic benefits. They also do not have the irritant effects of tea and coffee, and do not normally contain any caffeine. Drink them sweetened with a little honey, or freshened with a slice of lemon. Here are some of the best teas to try for various ailments:
■ Calming the nerves, inducing sleep: chamomile, limeflower, passion flower, red clover.
■ Infections or colds: rosehip, comfrey, aniseed, licorice, sage.
■ To improve liver function: agrimony, mugwort, angelica.
■ Indigestion or tummyache: peppermint, dill,

fennel, lemon grass, aniseed, lemon balm.
- As a tonic: nettle, mint, ginseng, rosemary, raspberry and strawberry leaf.
- Diuretics for weight loss and the kidneys: celery seed, dandelion, couchgrass, golden rod, agrimony.

You can also drink herbal teas for their flavour alone. Delicious blends are now available from most supermarkets and healthfood shops. Try them iced in summer: iced peppermint tea with lemon and fresh mint is a delicious option.

FRUIT AND VEGETABLE JUICES

Fresh fruit juice is considered to be the equivalent of a serving of fresh fruit. In fact, fresh fruit and vegetable juices are essential parts of cancer-protection diets. Raw juices do most of the things that solid raw foods do, but in a way that places minimum strain on the digestive system. The concentrated vitamins, minerals, trace elements, enzymes, sugars and proteins they contain are absorbed into the bloodstream almost as soon as they reach the stomach and small intestine.

If you are worried about the number of fresh vegetable and fruit servings you are getting throughout the week, consider purchasing a juicer and making your own fresh juices regularly. I love juicing and, although it might sound unappealing, my favourite juice is carrot and orange. It is such a quick, tasty, satisfying way to get a lot of goodness into your body. Try a glass of carrot and apple juice after a sleepless night and you will experience an astonishing energy boost.

CALORIE COUNTING

Counting calories is pretty much a thing of the past. When you concentrate on eating the right quantities of the right sorts of foods, based on the food pyramid, it's pretty unlikely that you will eat more than you need. The problem with calorie counting is that it fosters an obsession with food. You end up checking the content of everything you eat, and you are constantly adding up totals. First and foremost, the calorie content of most foods is an average content rather than the exact content so, try as you may, you will never meet your target exactly. Secondly, you may find that you choose foods with a low calorie content, rather than on the basis of their nutritional value. For example, you could, theoretically, eat five packets of low-fat crisps and drink several glasses of wine and still be within your calorie allocation for the day. What this fails to take

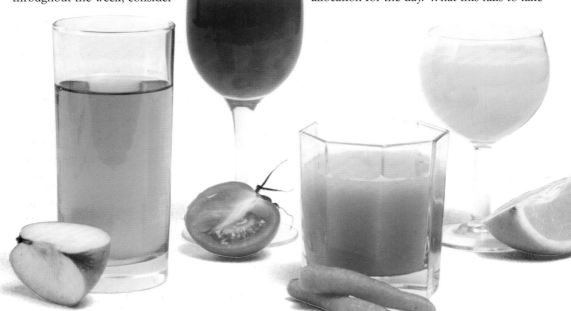

into consideration, however, is the fact that you have eaten nothing good for you.

Instead, the modern way of looking at diet involves organizing meals and snacks so that you get enough of the right kinds of food. If you are eating between five and ten servings of fruit and vegetables a day, as well as a bowl of pasta, a wholemeal sandwich and some lean meat or fish, you are unlikely to eat more than you should in terms of energy content. You also need to concentrate on ensuring that you don't eat too much fat, particularly the saturated kind.

It may, however, be useful to know roughly how many calories you should consume each day. If only to use it as a basis for figuring out how much fat, for example, you are eating, or what percentage of your diet is based on carbohydrates.

As we know, fat is broken down into 'saturated' and 'unsaturated'. Remember that your total fat intake for a day should be around 30 per cent of your total calorie intake – that's between 50 and 80 grams for most people.

If you eat this number of calories per day	Total saturated fat per day (grams)	Total fat intake per day (grams)
1,600	18 or less	53 or less
2,000	20 or less	65 or less
2,200	24 or less	73 or less
2,500	25 or less	80 or less

So, if a takeaway sandwich listed 12 g of fat, of which 8.8 were saturated, you would be consuming roughly a fifth of your fat intake for the day, and about a third of your saturated fat intake. As a guideline, the following number of calories are likely to be appropriate. Remember, however, that every body is different, as is every lifestyle.

Age	Males	Females
Young adults	2,500 (3,350 if very active)	2,150 (2,400 if pregnant; 2,750 if breastfeeding)
Middle-aged	2,400 (3,350 if very active)	1,900 (2,500 if very active)
Over 75	2,150	1,680

LOW-CALORIE DIETS

Just one pound of excess fat on the body is the equivalent of 3,500 calories consumed. In order to diet off that one pound of fat you must therefore create a negative energy balance of 3,500 calories. In terms of weight control by diet alone, that is a lot. For a woman whose average daily intake might be only about 2,000 calories, cutting 3,500 over the space of a few days brings her very close to the area where the body would regard itself as in starvation. With women there is not much margin – a drop of only about 500 calories per day would be enough in a slim woman for the onset of the starvation cycle. After ten days of relative starvation the body stops burning solely carbohydrate and fat and draws on protein from the muscles. This is the last thing you want, as it is your muscles which burn up energy.

BODY MASS INDEX

Body Mass Index, or BMI, is a measure of weight that is widely used by insurance companies, as a measure of your health. BMIs have replaced the traditional 'height-weight' charts, which simply didn't take into consideration different body sizes.

This is how it works:

- If your BMI is below 19, you are probably underweight. You may, however, have feather-light bones, in which case you might be fine. It's all relative.
- If your BMI is over 30, then you are overweight. However, as long as you take regular exercise and your hips are larger than your waist, your weight is probably nothing to worry about.
- If your BMI is more than about 35, you are definitely obese and, from a health point of view, it's something you should probably do something about.
- Ideally, your BMI should fall somewhere between 20 and 25, which would indicate that you are probably a healthy weight for your height.

Here's how to calculate it: BMI = $weight/height^2$

Sounds complicated? It isn't. Basically, you need

to divide your weight by your height, twice. Use a calculator and follow these instructions: Key in your weight (in kilograms). Press '÷' or '/'. Tap in your height (in metres). Press '÷' or '/' again. Tap in your height a second time. Press '='. The result is your BMI number.

■ So, let's say you weigh 64 kg, and you are 1·65 metres tall.

■ Your BMI number is: $64 \div 1.65 \div 1.65 = 23·5$

That's well within the healthy weight guidelines. So throw the standard height charts away. There is plenty of space for variation here, and as long as you look and feel good, you are at a weight that is right for you.

FINDING YOUR NATURAL WEIGHT

Diets are out – they do not work! I can't stress this strongly enough. Sure, anyone who starves themselves will lose weight. But remember, a good proportion of the weight you lose will be water (soon to return, when the diet is over), and you'll also trick your metabolism into believing you are starving, so it will slow down to conserve energy.

The negative effects of dieting are as follows:

■ It creates an unhealthy obsession with food. When you are constantly considering what you can and cannot eat, and depriving your body of what it really needs, you think about food constantly. When the diet is over, that obsession doesn't go away. In my younger days, whenever I denied myself a food type it would be literally all that I wanted to eat. In the end I would crave it so much that I would have to have it, then I would binge completely on it and end up feeling terrible and sick.

■ There is, unquestionably, a yo-yo effect. Dieters lose weight, but they do so not by changing eating habits, but through deprivation. Once again, as soon as the diet is over, you return to your old habits and the fat piles back on.

■ You slow down your metabolism to such a degree that when you do start eating normally, you put on weight because it is working that much more slowly. It naturally wants to lay down fat in case you should decide to starve it again.

■ You are more likely to binge-eat and then starve, which puts enormous strain on the body.

So what's the answer? It's simple, really. Think like a thin person. Change your eating habits completely and forget about your weight. If that sounds crazy, consider this:

Thin people forget to eat. It's true! They are not obsessed with food and they eat what they want when they are hungry. If you adopt the same attitude, you will find your natural weight. It will be a slow process, but give yourself a few months and you can expect to lose between a pound and two pounds every single week.

Freya Copeland
✿ I eat a Mediterranean diet and can recommend it as a tasty way to eat low-fat, healthy food. I eat loads of vegetables, fruit and pasta, and use olive oil in my cooking. As a vegetarian I find this type of diet keeps me from eating too much cheese, which I love but is laden with fat.

Thin people often eat a normal breakfast. They might have a craving for a sticky bun mid-morning. Dieters look on wistfully and opt for a cup of tea, or an apple. The slim person eats the sticky bun and, come lunch, probably feels fairly full and opts for a salad, or a sandwich. The dieter, on the other hand, is starving, and feeling very deprived. She might hold out through lunch (cottage cheese and an apple), but come mid-afternoon, the craving is too great and she eats not one sticky bun but two, and sneaks a packet of crisps as well. The thin person has an apple mid-afternoon, which gets her through to dinner. She's meeting up with friends, and doesn't think much about food. When mealtime rolls around, she's had a couple of canapés and a glass or two of wine. All she feels like now is a bowl of soup. But the dieter has wrecked her diet. I'll start again tomorrow, she says to herself, and proceeds to order a large pizza and drink a bottle of wine alongside. She wakes up feeling guilty, and resolves to have more will power, but the endless cycle starts again.

The message is this. If you eat normally, when you are hungry, you will find your natural weight. If you follow the food pyramid (see page 28), you'll be getting plenty of nutritious, healthy food and you will be less likely to suffer cravings. It's not easy to squeeze up to 10 servings of fruit and vegetables into a day, and when you've managed that, there isn't a whole lot of room left for anything else. Find inventive ways to eat well, and don't eat until you are hungry. If you crave something sweet, eat a little of what you feel like. The craving will be satisfied, and you won't be tempted to eat too much. If you are desperate for something fatty, go for it. Just try to eat smaller portions and savour every mouthful.

This is the way to lose weight without dieting and there is no question that it works. You'll find that when you are full and content, having eaten good food that tastes delicious, you won't need to eat so much, and you won't think about food all the time.

The following might help:

■ Drink a glass of freshly-squeezed grapefruit juice every morning to cleanse, help break down fats and suppress appetite.

■ Drink at least 1.5 l of fresh water each day, to help the body to flush out toxins and cleanse the digestive system, making it work more effectively.

■ Join an exercise class or find a form of exercise that you can fit into your lifestyle (see Chapter One).

■ Work on improving your self-esteem. Hold yourself properly. Wear clothes that fit. A good attitude can make you feel more energetic, which translates itself into an improved sense of well-being. Studies show that when you are feeling well, you are less hungry and tired – which -in turn may help you to lose unwanted pounds.

■ If you have trouble resisting food and always feel hungry, consider acupuncture, which can help you cope with cravings and food

addictions. Three or four sessions with a registered practitioner may tip the scales in your favour.

SUPPLEMENTS FOR WEIGHT LOSS

■ There is some evidence that bee pollen, which is available as a powder or in tablet form, may stimulate the metabolism and suppress the appetite, as well as boosting immunity. Don't use this if you are allergic to bee stings or honey.

■ Brewer's yeast may reduce cravings for sweet food.

■ The herb bladderwrack may help to encourage the metabolism. You can buy it in tablet form, or as a tincture (herbs suspended in alcohol). Take daily for best effects, but always follow dosage instructions.

■ A mild chromium deficiency may cause cravings and a drop in blood sugar. Take a supplement each day to even out blood sugar levels.

■ Acidophilus and other healthy bacteria can help to enhance digestion, which means that nutrients are better absorbed and waste is better eliminated.

■ Co-enzyme Q10 helps the body's cells use oxygen and generate energy. There is some evidence that people supplementing CoQ10 are able to lose weight more quickly. Take 15-30 mg daily.

EASY NUTRITION

It's not easy to juggle a busy lifestyle, and healthy eating is often the first thing to go when we are under stress. It does seem much easier to fill the freezer with ready-prepared meals, or to pick up a burger on the way home from work. These are habits that have to go – both for your long-term health, your weight and the way your body is able to cope with your day-to-day life.

■ Try to plan your meals in advance, and take a list to the supermarket. If you've got good food in the fridge, you are more likely to eat it.

■ Remember that it takes very little time to prepare a healthy meal – certainly no more than it does to heat up a pre-cooked meal.

Here are some ideas that will help you to eat according to the food pyramid, and find the time to prepare meals that will keep you going.

BREAKFAST

Try to eat a little breakfast if you can – it avoids blood sugar drops mid-morning which could make you reach for a doughnut or a chocolate bar to get you through to lunch. If you really can't bear the thought of breakfast, a glass of fruit juice will help to stave off hunger pangs. Remember that breakfast doesn't need to take place first thing in the morning. If you prefer, eat something when you arrive at work or mid-morning at your desk. You can now get milk and cereal 'instant' meals in a pot, which can be very useful if you are pressed for time in the mornings. Try one of the following:

- A banana, a glass of fresh orange or grapefruit juice and a piece of wholemeal toast.
- A bowl of muesli or other wholegrain cereal, with a little semi-skimmed milk and sliced bananas or strawberries.
- A hardboiled egg (cook it the night before), wholemeal toast and sliced tomatoes.
- Fresh fruit, topped with a dollop of Greek yoghurt and a little honey.
- A sandwich with boiled egg, a slice of lean ham, tomatoes and cucumber.

LUNCH

There is still a lurking belief that lunch has to be hot to be nutritious. In fact, studies show quite the opposite. A fresh sandwich, with some salad on wholegrain bread, is just as nutritious as a hot meal, and apart from being less fattening, it will also prevent that mid-afternoon energy dip that occurs after eating a large meal. It is undoubtedly better to eat your main meal at lunchtime, giving your body time to digest it while you are active rather than asleep, but a main meal doesn't need to be cooked to be nutritious. After a good nutritious lunch, you'll find that you are less hungry at dinnertime, and much less likely to snack in the afternoons. Here are some suggestions:

- Wholegrain bread sandwich, with tuna, sweetcorn, peppers and salad. Fresh juice and a piece of fruit.
- Greek salad, with feta cheese, cucumbers, tomatoes, olives and a light dressing. Have a wholegrain bun on the side and a piece of fruit for dessert.
- A bowl of soup – cold or hot – with a wholegrain roll, a good-sized piece of cheese and fruit salad for dessert.
- Couscous salad with roasted vegetables. Choose a glass of fresh juice on the side, and a yoghurt or a piece of fruit for dessert.
- Pasta lightly cooked with a tomato sauce. Add a glass of fresh juice and a small crunchy green salad and you've got a perfect meal. Try adding a few prawns to the sauce for extra nutrition and flavour.
- Pizza with a thin crust, lots of fresh vegetables and only a sprinkling of cheese. If you have time to make your own, use feta and parmesan cheese for a lower fat alternative instead of cheddar or mozzarella, or use a strong tasting cheddar so you'll need less.
- Beans on toast.
- A bagel with low-fat cheese and lots of salad.
- Peanut butter on wholemeal bread.
- Pitta bread filled with cottage cheese, spring onions and prawns.
- Salad with tuna, olives, lettuce, green beans, tomatoes and anchovies.

SNACKS

If you find you're hungry between meals, don't try to ignore the feeling. Try one of these snacks to fill the gap.

- Pretzels – they are low in fat. Try to choose a low-salt brand.
- Chop some fresh carrots, cucumber, sugar-snap peas and dwarf sweetcorn in advance and keep them in a glass of chilled water in the fridge. Dip them in some low-fat humus or tsatziki.
- A handful of pistachios, which are less fattening than some other nuts.
- Air-popped popcorn sprinkled with a little sea-salt – almost no fat!
- Cottage cheese sprinkled with black pepper, on crispbread.
- A bowl of cereal with a little milk.

DINNER

Dinnertime has become later and later, as we work longer hours and wait for partners to return home. This has a fairly dramatic effect on both weight and sleep. Heavy meals, eaten late in the day, are not burned off as quickly as meals eaten earlier in the day. The later you eat, the worse the effect. Also, going to bed on a full stomach can mean a less restful sleep, as your body copes with digesting rather than relaxing and rejuvenating. What's the answer? Try to eat your main meal earlier in the day. If that's impossible, eat something substantial soon after you get home from work, and if you have to be sociable at the dinner table later in the evening, pick at a salad, or sip a cup of soup. Try to stick to the 6 o'clock rule – nothing but snacks or light meals should be eaten after that time. I know countless people who have lost kilos in weight simply by changing their eating habits to fit in with this rule.

- Stir-fry a chicken breast that you've marinated the night before. You can either buy a good marinade, or make-your own. Make sure you use a little olive oil, something acidic, like lemon juice or vinegar, and then add anything that appeals. Try garlic and rosemary, honey and lemon, coriander and lime, or even coconut milk with lemongrass and coriander. Add some crunchy peppers, green beans and thinly sliced carrots to the pan and season to taste.
- Add cooked chicken breast to a pitta stuffed with cucumber and tomato wedges, salad and a dollop of tsatziki.
- Place a piece of salmon or tuna in some foil with a squirt of lemon, a sprig of parsley and a few spring onions and bake for about 15 minutes. Serve with a salad of lettuce and raw vegetables, topped with a light French dressing. Add a wholegrain roll. Or, if you have time, a baked potato.
- Make a lasagne with fresh vegetable sauce from the supermarket, fresh lasagne leaves, cottage cheese and parmesan. Spread the layers with sauce, add a few chopped mushrooms, onions, tomatoes or whatever takes your fancy, then spread with cottage cheese. Repeat the layers then cover with grated parmesan cheese. Bake for about 25–30 minutes at 190°C/375°F/Gas 5.
- Roast a chicken at the weekend, and you can serve it in a variety of ways during the week. Add a little to cooked pasta topped with some grated cheese, steamed broccoli and sweetcorn. Or make a chicken salad with orange slices, cucumbers, sugar-snap peas, lettuce, sweetcorn and sliced apples in a French dressing.
- Ready-cooked rice is a good bet – look in the freezer section of your supermarket. Use it as a basis for a rice salad, with lots of roasted vegetables such as peppers, courgettes, fennel and onions. Add a little feta cheese and Greek dressing for flavour. Or stir fry rice with lightly cooked vegetables and a little ham.
- Grill a lamb or pork chop with a dash of balsamic vinegar or Worcestershire sauce. Serve with potatoes (baked or boiled) and seasoned with a little sea salt and some black pepper, and some lightly steamed broccoli, courgettes and sweetcorn on the side.

DESSERTS

- Fresh fruit.
- Frozen yoghurt with maple syrup, raisins and walnuts.
- Baked apples with raisins and yoghurt.
- Baked bananas with a little rum and brown sugar. Serve with Greek yoghurt.
- Fruit crumble and custard made with skimmed milk.
- Organic ice cream with fresh strawberries or other fruits in season
- Fresh fruits, such as mango, strawberries, kiwis, blueberries, plums and nectarines in a little orange juice and a teaspoon of brown sugar. Add a dash of orange liqueur for extra flavour.
- Fruit salad with grated dark chocolate on top.
- A low-fat chocolate brownie, piled high with strawberries and other fruit in season.

VITAMINS AND MINERALS IN FOOD

Eating the right foods doesn't necessarily mean that you are getting enough nutrients. Refining and processing foods takes out much of the nutritional value – before our food ever reaches the supermarket it may be nutritionally deficient. Therefore, take extra steps to preserve the nutritional content of your food whenever possible:

- Eat the skins of vegetables whenever possible.
- Don't cut, wash or soak fruit and vegetables until you are ready to eat them. Exposing their cut surfaces to air reduces many nutrients.
- Eat brown, unpolished rice and whole grains.
- Choose fresh fruit and vegetables first, but remember that nutritional value decreases with age. Frozen is a better option if you aren't going to eat the food immediately.
- Eat raw whenever possible; if cooking, use as little water as possible.
- If you do boil fruit or vegetables, use the cooking water for sauces or gravy.
- Eat organic food whenever possible. It may be a little more expensive, but you can be sure that what you are eating has been grown without the use of pesticides and other chemicals.

IS A GOOD DIET EXPENSIVE?

A good diet doesn't need to be expensive, and it is quite likely to be cheaper than a poor diet. Few people, for instance, need to eat expensive things like meat every day (vegetable proteins, such as lentils and tofu, are cheap in comparison), and fresh foods are always much cheaper than ready-prepared, refined foods. Your main problem may be finding the time to buy fresh food several times a week, then to cook and eat properly, but that can be overcome with a little organisation. Take time to make a big, fresh vegetable stew or soup with plenty of pulses and lightly cooked vegetables. If you freeze it in small quantities as soon as it is prepared, you will have a nutritious meal on hand when time is tight. Rice and pulses can also be cooked and prepared in large batches and frozen. If you are pressed for time, you may want to go for pre-prepared salads. These might be a little more expensive, but you are more

Kevin Pallister
✿ *I am a vegetarian and find the most nutritional, low fat and tasty alternative to meat is Quorn – and I eat a lot of it. My favourite way of cooking it is in a stir-fry with a little olive oil and a black-bean sauce and loads of fresh mixed veg.*

likely to use them if they are easy to access, rather than throwing out wilted lettuce that you haven't got round to washing and preparing.

BOOSTING YOUR IMMUNE SYSTEM

The immune system is crucial, protecting the body from invaders such as cancer cells, bacteria, viruses, parasites and fungi and ensuring that you recover from illness quickly and efficiently. A healthy immune system is vital for overall health, and there are a number of nutritional elements that will help to keep it strong, and functioning well.

Your immune system can become impaired by the following factors:

- injuries
- surgery
- the overuse of antibiotics, which can suppress the immune system, and destroy the healthy bacteria of the bowel, called flora
- some drugs
- digestive disorders, like candida, enzyme deficiencies and chronic constipation
- poor diet
- pollution
- stress
- genetic problems
- disease
- inherited weaknesses.

Here's what to do:

- Ensure that you get plenty of sleep.
- Drink lots of fresh, plain water, which helps to cleanse the system.
- Get plenty of exercise.
- Eat a balanced diet, rich in whole foods, nuts and seeds, fresh vegetables and fruit, high in fibre, low in saturated fat, and avoid smoking, environmental pollutants, too

much alcohol, saturated fats, refined grains and sweeteners, all of which compromise immune activity.

- Take a good multi-vitamin and mineral supplement to ensure that you have adequate quantities of nutrients with immune-boosting activity. These include vitamin A, B-complex, C, E and the minerals zinc and selenium.

HEALTHY SHOPPING

Base your shopping on fresh foods as far as possible, but remember that food doesn't need to be expensive or exotic to be nutritious.

- Check the fat content and buy lower fat choices. Watch out for foods that have been over-processed, or that contain saturated fats (see page 19).
- Put fruit and vegetables at the top of your shopping list. Vegetables, especially those in season, are the most economical choice. Colour is a good guide. The dark green and orange coloured fruits and vegetables are the richest sources of vitamins A, C and E, which are the antioxidants (see page 26). Add these to your shopping trolley regularly.
- Root vegetables have very little waste and can be stored for a longer time than green, leafy vegetables. Store them in a dark,

cool place to keep them fresh.
- Frozen vegetables and fruit are very convenient and just as nourishing as fresh. It is best to pick up frozen vegetables and fruit last, so that you can get them to the freezer more quickly.

SUPER SEASONING

Seasonings can make a bland meal into something special. Experiment with herbs, spices and other exotic seasonings to make your food more delicious without adding unnecessary fat or calories.

- Use black pepper more often as an alternative flavouring to salt.
- Buy garlic, ginger and onion to add flavour to cooked dishes.
- Use spices more often to reduce the amount of salt you add to cooked dishes such as casseroles and curries. Many herbs and spices have therapeutic benefits, and will enhance the digestive process, among other things. Most herbs are nutritious, and will improve the nutritional value of your meal as well as adding flavour. The more flavourful a meal, the more satisfying it can be.
- Add herbs, fresh or dried to salads and cooked meals.
- Try to buy fresh herbs, which retain more of their nutritional value as well as being more flavourful. Potted herb plants, such as parsley or basil, cost only a little more than ready-cut packets and last longer. Most supermarkets now supply several herbs in one package: for example, Thai or Indian fresh herbs and spices, or Italian or Greek. Be adventurous!

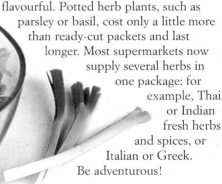
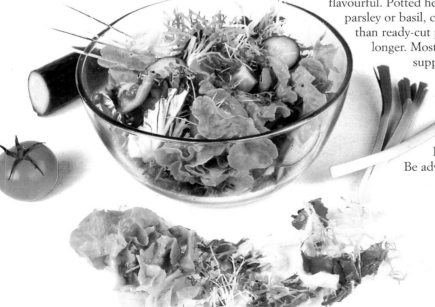

3. Rest and relaxation

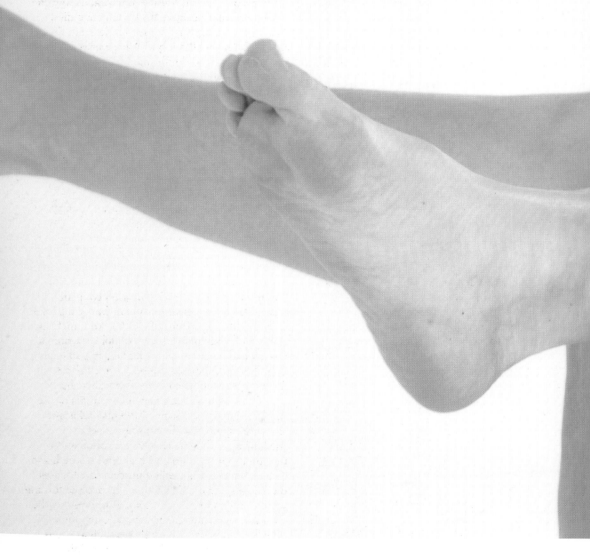

I T'S EASY TO get caught up in the chaos of daily life, and time for ourselves is often low on the list of priorities. The problem is that on the surface we appear to manage. We get through hectic days that stretch into weeks and, although we feel tired and out of sorts, we do somehow keep all the balls in the air. It's only when we stop – say, on holiday – that we realize how completely exhausted we are. That's often the time that we start to readjust our priorities. There's more to life than the rat race, and if we don't find time for ourselves, a very important part of the holistic equation is missing. Holistic health means all-round health – that's mind, body and spirit. We might eat well and get some

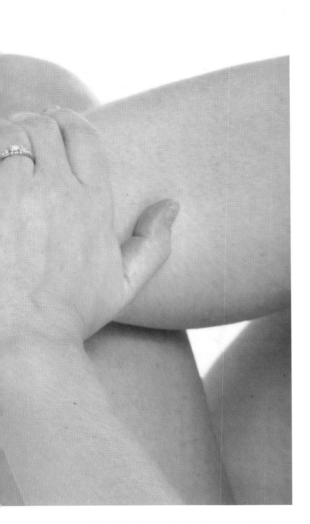

emotional and physical – that we just cannot replace. And then there's the spiritual angle. You don't have to believe in any religion to understand the concept of spirit. Spirit is our vital energy, the force that keeps us alive. When someone dies, that energy disappears. Some people claim they can feel it leaving the room. Whatever you believe, there is no doubt that we have an inner energy that is responsible for life. There is also no doubt that spirit needs peace to survive.

Paula Tilbrook

✿ *When I have a day off, I really treasure it and try to do as little as possible, so I can relax as much as possible.*

✿ *Each day I do five minutes' worth of breathing exercises to combat hypertension. I sit in a quiet room and breathe deeply using my diaphragm; this really relaxes and centres me.*

That's where rest and relaxation come in. Relaxation is not, as you probably know, achieved by sitting down in front of the TV. You might be stopping the action, but you are doing nothing to lower the adrenaline that is raging around your body. This form of passive relaxation has no therapeutic benefits and does little apart from take the weight off your feet. The stresses of the day, the criticisms, disappointments and anger stay locked in the body, causing anxiety, frustration, and depression in the mind, and tension in the muscles and ligaments of the body. True relaxation is a healing process that focuses on relaxing the mind and body. It involves turning your attention inwards to control and resolve the effects of stress rather than suppressing those effects with short-term measures such as drugs, cigarettes and alcohol. Relaxation is a skill. Practised correctly it is an important factor in preventing disease on every level, from the general feeling of ease and well-being which increases when adrenaline levels are lowered to fighting off the common cold and even reducing the risk of developing life-threatening illnesses.

Once again, however, we are back to the same old problem. How do we fit it in?

exercise. All right, that's the body covered. But what about our minds and spirits?

Eventually, overdoing it on any front will lead to mental exhaustion. When we cannot cope emotionally, our physical health will suffer. The mind – body relationship is incredibly strong, and when things start to slip emotionally, there's a domino effect. We use up resources – both

LEISURE TIME

Leisure plays an important role in overall health and well-being. If you don't get enough of it, you can begin to feel irritable, fatigued and depressed. Over time, life without leisure can lead to ulcers, migraines, cardiovascular disease, high blood pressure and other physical ailments.

Leisure activities can help you to feel more satisfied with your life, as well as making you feel more energized and excited to wake up in the morning.

According to studies, most Westerners have difficulty creating leisure time and using it properly. Leisure tends to be task-orientated, demand-orientated and pressurized. Instead of experiencing the joy and playfulness of leisure, people put themselves at risk of draining energy reserves even further. Leisure is the time to renew yourself and is as essential as sleeping, exercising and eating properly.

Alyson Spiro

✿ To relieve tension I put a few drops of lavender oil in my bath water and take a long luxurious bath. I come out feeling like a new person!

✿ If one of my children is poorly I always put some lavender oil on their pillow at night before putting them to bed. It is very soothing and induces sleep.

CREATING LEISURE

It takes effort and planning to work enjoyable activities into your life. Set aside time each day for a leisure activity you enjoy, even if it is just a ten-minute walk around the block, or a warm bath with a book in hand. Find a reason to make room in your life for leisure. It might be as simple as telling yourself that you want to live longer, or have a better relationship with your spouse, children or friends. Whatever it is, it has to be something that is more important to you than work. If it's not, you are unlikely to stick with it.

Most people have more free time than they think. How you spend it is the problem, experts say. On average, Westerners have about 41 hours of free time a week when they are not working, doing household chores or sleeping. But because the number of leisure activities is expanding, the amount of time we can devote to any one activity is shrinking. One activity, watching television, does take precedence over all others. One study found that over 30 per cent of our leisure time is spent in front of the television. In comparison, socializing and reading, the second and third most popular activities, accounted for only eight and six per cent respectively of the available leisure time each day.

The key to a healthy and rejuvenating leisure life is to participate in a variety of stimulating activities. Experts recommend the following approach for people who want to spend their time doing better things:

- Keep a diary. For a week, write down what you are doing every 30 minutes, including things like cooking and working. At the end of the week take a look at your diary and see how much time you spent working and how much free time you had. Each day, rate your satisfaction with each leisure activity. If you are filling your time with obligations you don't find rewarding, you should make changes.
- Set limits. It is important to draw boundaries between your work and home life. For example, avoid taking work home at night. Dr Jeanne Murrone, a clinical psychologist, says, 'By doing that you are letting both your employer and your family know that your leisure time is just as important to you as getting to work on time, meeting your deadlines and whatever else you do on the job.'
- Create space. Create time for yourself at the end of the day, even if it is only 15 or 20 minutes, to be alone with your thoughts. This helps to make the transition between work and home. Walking, reading the newspaper or even changing clothes can have the same effect.
- Make your own fun. Know yourself and what you think is entertaining and rewarding. Make a list of your strengths and weaknesses: what you like to do and what you don't. Then make your leisure choice based on that list.

■ Be imperfect. Some people avoid doing certain leisure activities because they don't feel that they can master them. It's important to recognize that you don't have to do everything well.

COPING WITH STRESS

Medical scientists divide people's behaviour into two types, depending on their reactions to stress. People with type A behaviour are competitive, ambitious and desperate to achieve. They always appear impatient, even aggressive, hurried and conscious of the time, and constantly seek to exert control over their environment. Type B people may be just as ambitious as those of type A, but they are more patient, easy going and relaxed. A type B personality would, for instance, look at a traffic jam as a positive experience. Things are beyond their control, they are in a car with a radio and have been given a space of time in which to relax. Type A personalities set themselves unrealistic targets and find it difficult to fit work into an allotted time. This type of behaviour develops partly as a result of upbringing and childhood experiences, and it is neither healthy nor productive. All the evidence suggests that people who are constantly stressed, and react aggressively to it, are more likely to develop heart disease or another serious illnesses and that, despite working excessive hours, they ultimately achieve little more than those whose working patterns are more balanced. Even people who are inherently stressed can learn to alter their beliefs, attitudes and habits to enjoy a better quality and quantity of life.

Although a link between stress and cancer is uncertain, some experts believe there is a type-C personality – one who is cancer prone because of chronic stress. A recent study shows that stress is one of the leading causes of many forms of cancer. Controlling stress may be the first step to preventing cancer, which can be considered to be a profound breakdown of health at all levels.

Behaviour modification involves learning about oneself and then practising drills to change from being stressed to being a calmer person. Some of the keys to making these changes include:

■ Stop rushing and living by the clock.
■ Concentrate on finishing one job at a time.
■ Learn to wait patiently when you have to, and make constructive use of your time while waiting.
■ Try to avoid situations that you find irritating.
■ Do not set yourself unnecessary deadlines, and avoid filling your diary with back-to-back appointments.
■ Stop becoming angry about things over which you have no control.
■ Learn to relax.
■ Create a life-plan, and find an extra hour or two each week to tackle things you have been putting off, or use that time for something pleasant.
■ Set aside 30 minutes every day for yourself.
■ Establish your priorities, and make sure that what is important to you is at the top of the list.

Sheree Murphy
✿ *If I cannot sleep at night, I reach for a book and read until my eyelids feel as if they are going to close, then, nine times out of ten, I will drop straight off. This is so much better than tossing and turning and fighting to get to sleep, which never works.*

SUPER STRESS MANAGEMENT

If you counted the number of times a day that people complained of being stressed, you'd probably hit 20 or 30 easily. It's got to be the most common complaint of our modern age, and 'being stressed' has become another way of saying tired, run-down or even just unhappy. Stress isn't all bad – if we didn't face some challenges, we'd probably sit around like lizards in the sun all day long. Too much stress, however, and we can suffer from health complaints that range from reduced immunity to nervous habits. Common symptoms include:

■ headaches
■ fatigue
■ niggling digestive disorders

- skin problems
- intolerant behaviour – perhaps flying off the handle at things that you would normally take in your stride.

BUT WHAT EXACTLY IS STRESS?

Stress is not actually an illness, but a response by the body to anything that puts a strain upon it. Most of us think of tense situations and worries as being the cause of stress. In reality, stresses can be far more profound and wide-ranging, and can include environmental stresses such as pollution, noise, housing problems, cold or too much heat; physical stresses, such as illness, injury, or an inadequate diet or one that is too high in refined foods, additives or toxins such as alcohol or caffeine; and mental stresses such as relationship problems, financial strains, job difficulties, and more.

All these factors have an effect on the body, causing it to make a series of rapid physiological changes, called 'adaptive responses', to deal with threatening or demanding situations.

In the first stage of stress, hormones are poured into the bloodstream. The pulse quickens, the lungs take in more oxygen to fuel the muscles, blood sugar increases to supply added energy, digestion slows, and perspiration increases.

In the second stage of stress, the body begins to repair the damage caused by the first stage. If the stressful situation is resolved, the stress symptoms vanish. If the stressful situation continues, however, a third stage, exhaustion, sets in, and the body's energy wears out. This stage may continue until vital organs are affected, and then disease or even death can result.

WHAT'S THE ANSWER?

Relaxation and exercise. Centuries ago, people might wrestle with a bear or a panther in a stressful situation. The adrenaline surging

around their bodies would be dispersed naturally, or they would meet with a grisly end. Today, we face different, but no less demanding stresses. And the worst thing is that they are around us all the time. We live by clocks, we race to and from work, school runs and shopping trips; our environment is noisy; we eat foods that place our bodies under even more pressure and then we expect it to be sorted by a couple of hours in front of the box with a drink in hand. Our bodies aren't designed that way. We need space to breathe, peace to relax and exercise to help disperse some of the adrenaline that hits fever pitch for the majority of our waking hours.

Paul Loughran
✿ *I practised the Alexander technique for four years at Drama College. These days, in order to relax, I put on some classical music, lie on the floor and try to clear all thoughts from my head. I find this has two benefits: my back and body become much less tense; my mind is clear and I can sleep much better. This is great because for years I slept very badly, which would affect my concentration at work.*

There are dozens of 'new' complementary therapies and remedies that can help to deal with the stresses of daily living (see page 47), but there are things that we can do on a practical, day-to-day level, to help ease the strain on our minds, bodies and, of course, spirits. We've already discussed making time for relaxation and rest, and we'll discuss the importance of good, restful sleep on page 50. Here are a couple of tricks I've learned to help me keep my cool. Try working out similar solutions to the situations that regularly wind you up.

TEN SAVING SECONDS

First and foremost in any stressful situation, count to ten. Ten seconds is the amount of time that it takes for an adrenaline surge to bottom out. When you feel an overwhelming urge to land a right-hook on your partner's cheek when he asks what's for dinner five seconds after you've walked through the door, or when your children have pushed you to breaking point, stop. Count to ten and then deal with the situation as calmly as you can.

Something that really used to stress me out

was the phone ringing when I'd just sat down to dinner, or was trying to get an early night – why does it always ring then? These days I don't give it the chance – I turn the phone off if I don't want to be disturbed.

Another thing that stresses me out is when I'm in a rush and everywhere I go there is a queue, whether it's in a bank, post office, petrol station or supermarket. Everyone seems to be conspiring to hold me up, and it really gets me wound up – I'm a type A person! I am getting better at coping with this situation – I just don't try any more to fit too much into half an hour. If there is a huge queue at the bank and I have five minutes to get to a meeting, I'll leave the bank and go back later. It's just not worth getting grey hairs for!

Some stress is healthy and invigorating, but too much can harm you. In order to be able to cope with stress, our bodies need to be as healthy and as strong as they can be. Complementary therapies are an excellent way of dealing with stress, primarily because they deal with you holistically. Here are some of the best stress-busters:

AROMATHERAPY

Essential oils are excellent for stress-reduction because many of them work on the nervous system and the brain to relax and soothe. Other oils are uplifting, which can be invaluable in times of serious stress. Massage with aromatherapy oils is very comforting, particularly because of the physical element of touch, and a few drops of essential oil in the bath can offer an opportunity to wash away the problems of the day while experiencing the benefits of the oil. Suitable oils include:

● Basil	● Geranium	● Neroli
● Chamomile	● Lavender	● Rose

Oils which strengthen the adrenal system, which is weakened by stress, include:

● Rosemary	● Ginger	● Lemongrass

LEARN TO RELAX
- Yoga may help to relieve stress and tension (see page 49), and stretching the body will ease muscle tension and teach you to breathe more efficiently.
- Biofeedback and meditation are also excellent relaxation therapies, and can be used in everyday life.
- Breathing is extremely important in controlling stress, and you can take special classes designed to teach you to breathe properly, releasing stress and tension.

BACK TO NATURE
- Herbs that encourage relaxation and act as a tonic to the nervous system include balm, lavender, chamomile, verbena, passiflora and oats. Any of these can be drunk as an infusion – as often as necessary in stressful situations.
- Ginseng is an excellent 'adaptogenic' herb, which means that it lifts you when you are tired, and relaxes you when you are stressed. It also works on the immune system and, energizes. Some therapists recommend that you take it daily in stressful times.

Other useful therapies include reflexology, which improves energy levels and helps us to relax.

The best advice, however, is to think positively and to allow yourself to be fallible. Even great achievers have failings, and we all need time to stop and take stock of our situations. Relax, treat your body with kindness. Best of all, enjoy life. That soon translates itself into a marvellous sense of well-being which leaves you feeling great.

MASSAGE

Massage can be used either to soothe and relax or to stimulate and revitalize. It is particularly effective for any stress-related and digestive disorders, and its gentle healing properties are equally effective for ailments ranging from a baby's colic through to the painful arthritic joints of the elderly. Even if you don't suffer from any of these problems, massage can enhance your sense of well-being.

Anyone can benefit from the healing effects of massage. The mere act of touch itself, combined with a caring attitude, will be immensely therapeutic. Obviously there are times and situations where an in-depth massage would be inappropriate or just too exhausting: a gentle hand massage or a simple face massage using the lightest of strokes can serve to soothe and relax.

Here's an easy massage that can be performed on people of all ages to soothe and relax.

For many the neck and shoulder are common areas of soreness and tension. Working these parts of the body can help you to ease these symptoms, which can, in turn, help the whole body to relax.

- Position yourself at your partner's head with her lying on her back.
- Oil the front of her body, starting with hands on the upper chest, then move down over the breastbone, out around the ribcage and back up the sides of the body to the starting position.
- Place hands on upper chest, fingers pointing toward each other and press down, gliding the hands out toward the top of the arm.
- Cradle the head in one hand and turn it slightly toward the left.
- With the other hand, glide firmly out from the centre of the chest to the top of the arm, back along the top of the shoulder and up the back of the neck to the base of the skull.
- Make little circles along the back of the neck to release tension, then continue back down the side of the neck to the chest.
- Stroke firmly down the side of the neck and out along the top of the shoulder, stretching the neck muscles.
- Turn head back to centre with both hands supporting the head under the neck, and pull gently to stretch out the neck muscles.
- Turn the head to the opposite side and repeat the sequence for the other shoulder.
- Return head to centre and pull gently once more.
- Make small overlapping, circular movements up the back of the neck to the skull and then stroke up the back of the head and off.
- Gently lower the head.

MEDITATION

Meditation is an ancient discipline that involves contemplation by focusing your mind on a thought or an object. It is a practice that can help you to understand everything in your life more clearly. It is a way of getting to know yourself that can transform and reveal your life in a new perspective. It will benefit you as a whole person. Among other things, it promotes physical relaxation and calm, which is good for your heart and cardiovascular system. When you meditate, your brain waves are in a different state from those of either waking or sleeping and both sides of your brain are active. The main purpose of meditation is to unite your mind and body, and in this way you will be able to find peace. People who meditate regularly claim that it makes their lives more full and active, with less stress and anxiety, and more restful and refreshing sleep.

A simple way to meditate is as follows:

- Sit quietly in a comfortable position and silently repeat a word or phrase while passively disregarding other thoughts. If your mind strays, acknowledge the other thoughts, but let them go, gently guiding yourself back to your word or phrase.
- Choose a word like 'calm', 'peace', or 'god' – if you are religious. It should be easy to pronounce and short enough to say silently as you exhale.
- Practise this kind of meditation for 20 minutes twice a day, and you will enjoy periods of stillness and quiet in your mind.

RELAXATION AND VISUALIZATION

Relaxation can slow heart rate, lower blood pressure and regulate breathing and metabolic rate. It also reduces adrenaline levels and allows the immune system to function more efficiently.

Visualization is the conscious use of the imagination to create images which can be used to heal or change aspects of your life. You need to be relaxed to be able to visualize, but, used well, it can help to deepen the relaxation process and overcome many of the mental and emotional problems that can lead to ill health. Some relaxation therapists encourage people to relieve serious health problems, including cancers, by imagining their medication destroying the disease process and visualizing the body using its healing powers to recover.

Therapists use and teach a number of different types of physical and mental (see visualization, above) relaxation techniques and in some cases induce very deep relaxation.

PHYSICAL RELAXATION

■ Active muscular relaxation: in this exercise, you tense your muscles and then release them to feel the physical and mental release that accompanies each movement. You will be taught how to work around your body, possibly starting with an arm or leg and focusing on every detail including fingers and toes. A therapist can guide you around your body, asking you to hold various muscles for about ten seconds. At the end of the session, which usually lasts for 20–30 minutes, she will tell you that the session is ending and when you open your eyes and stretch you will feel relaxed and refreshed.

■ Passive muscular relaxation is similar to tense-release, but instead of tensing a muscle group you focus your attention on the group, acknowledge the tension already held there and then release it. You may be asked to imagine a slow wave of relaxation washing through the muscles, lengthening and expanding them, loosening any points of tension.

MENTAL RELAXATION

■ Visualization often involves creating an imaginary place. When you are relaxed and lying with your eyes closed, the therapist will tell you to retreat in your mind to a special place, such as a cosy bed or a desert island. She will encourage you to use all your senses to explore the place, talking slowly in order to give you time to create the scene. When you have established your special place in your mind, your mind should be relaxed, and be receptive to anything you tell it. This would be the point where affirmations (positive statements) would be fed to you – such as, 'I am a calm and confident person. I can cope with stress in this or that way. . .'

YOGA FOR RELAXATION

Yoga can alleviate many of the problems we face today. The postures keep the body free of tension and the emphasis on breathing keeps the emotional body balanced and clear. When you practise yoga, the body is gently and skilfully manoeuvred in all directions. Consequently every muscle is stretched and toned. The internal organs are massaged, squeezed and expanded, improving their general function. The skeletal system is flexed, extended, rotated and twisted, creating greater joint mobility. The spine is encouraged to maintain a healthy, upright and pain-free condition. The circulation is improved. The breathing capacity and elasticity of the lungs are enhanced. The endocrine system is balanced and the nervous system soothed and stimulated to allow maximum efficiency. Movements performed are mirrored on both sides of the body to create perfect balance. Ultimately, your body becomes like 'an instrument' that you can learn to play and finely tune. You learn to respond to your body's needs, adapting and controlling as necessary in order to maintain perfect health.

You may wish to join a yoga class, and there are some designed for people of all ages and levels of fitness that focus on relaxation and

Steve Magan
❀ *Believe in the art of the possible: do not set your aims and goals in life too high, then you won't stress yourself out so much if you can't achieve them.*
❀ *If you cant rest or sleep, try a 'Steve Magan Power Nap'. I was once working flat out on a TV show from 6am until 5pm, then rushing off to do an evening performance of* Blood Brothers *in the West End. I never got a break, so when I got to the theatre, I used to go to a quiet room, turn off the lights and for 30–40 minutes do absolutely nothing. I used to concentrate on slowing down my breathing, clearing my mind and relaxing every muscle in my body. It is almost like self-hypnosis and it really calms and relaxes me. Give it a try as a pick-me-up.*

breathing, as well as whole-body fitness and well-being.

STRESS-BUSTERS

■ Laugh! Studies have shown that stress-fighting brain chemicals are released when you laugh, and experts claim that a good laugh relaxes tense muscles, speeds more oxygen into your system and lowers your blood pressure. There is even some indication that a smile is all that is necessary to ignite a positive mood.

■ Downshift. Living beyond your means can make you ill. One researcher studied British census data on 8,000 households and found that families trying to maintain lifestyles they couldn't afford were likely to have health problems.

■ Say no. Stressed people often cannot assert themselves. Instead of doing things you don't want to do, or don't have time to do, be a little selfish and say no for a change. People will respect you for your honesty, and you'll feel a lot better for making a statement instead of suppressing a whole heap of negative feelings.

■ Make lists. Learn to prioritize. At the start of every day, pick the single most important task to complete and then finish it. If you are a person who already makes a 'to-do list', never write one with more than five items. That way, you're more likely to get all the things done and you'll feel a greater sense of accomplishment and control. When you've finished one list, go ahead and make another five-item list.

THE IMPORTANCE OF SLEEP

It's not cool to admit to needing too much sleep. Margaret Thatcher, for example, slept for only a few hours a night and ran a country. We are spending an increasing number of hours in the office and our society continues to spread the myth that the tougher you are, the less sleep you need. It's not surprising that we are, as a nation, getting sicker and suffering more stress. Sleep is essential, and here's why:

■ Sleep maximizes the quality of our lives. When you sleep better, you feel better. You are more likely to perform at optimal levels and to maintain other healthy behaviours, like exercise and good diet.

■ The body releases its greatest concentration of growth hormone – the stuff that helps to strengthen the body and repair damaged tissues – during sleep.

■ Studies have shown that there is a close connection between sleep and the immune system. Sleep-deprived people seem to experience a decrease in the activity of natural killer cells and other immune system goodies that keep the body healthy and infection free.

■ Sleep has a reactivating effect on the central nervous system and the brain. Without sleep, neither functions at its maximum capacity.

■ Lack of sleep can lead to poor memory, the inability to make reasoned decisions or to concentrate, as well as irritability and, of course, fatigue.

HOW MUCH SLEEP DO YOU REALLY NEED?

If you feel that you get less sleep than you need, you are not alone. More people complain about sleep than any other single health issue.

Malandra Burrows
✿ *A good night out on the town with my girlfriends is a great stress buster. Work hard and play hard is my philosophy.*

Eight hours is probably the average requirement, but sleep needs, like everything else, are completely individual. About two-thirds of us get between six and a half and eight and a half hours every night. Just over 15 per cent of us sleep for more than that, and about the same sleep for less than six hours and feel just fine. 'Normal' is that which is correct for you, and every person differs in their sleep requirements.

There's no point in fighting your body clock. If you lie awake at night counting sheep, doze in

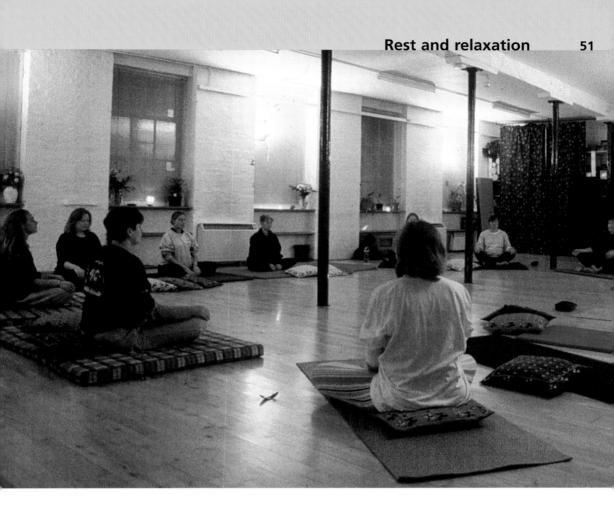

and out of sleep for the remainder of the night and feel like death the next morning, you probably need less than you think you do. Try going to bed an hour or two later, or wait until you are really tired. If that doesn't happen until well past the witching hour, maybe you are one of the minority of people who can get by – indeed, thrive – on less than five hours a night. Try to find a pattern that works for you. If you are tired, go to bed. Don't lie around in bed reading and listening to music. Go to bed only when you feel sleepy, read if that helps you get off to sleep, and then turn off the light the minute you feel your eyelids drop. Try a few days without setting the alarm. Go to bed at your normal hour and wake up naturally. You'll soon see a pattern emerging, and the number of hours you naturally sleep are probably the number of hours of sleep you really need.

CATNAPS AND POWER SNOOZES

In many cultures, an afternoon sleep, or siesta, is the norm, and there is evidence to suggest that an afternoon nap that does not interfere with night sleep can improve your mood, concentration and productivity. One Swedish study showed that a 25-minute nap (no longer, because you'll slip into a deeper sleep that will be difficult to wake up from) can be enormously restorative, particularly after a difficult night. If you are feeling tired, give in and lie down. Set an alarm so you don't sleep for longer than the recommended maximum. Shiftworkers or people who work at home may find it easier to fit in a nap, but if you work in an office, don't give up. Plenty of people have learned the benefits of 'powernaps' and have trained themselves to drop off, with head on desk, in the middle of a busy office or in the corner of the canteen over the lunch hour. If a nap works for you, find a way to take one.

INSUFFICIENT SLEEP OR INADEQUATE NUTRITION

Fatigue doesn't necessary relate to the amount of sleep you have had. Doctors report that one of the most common problems they see in their surgeries on a daily basis is chronic fatigue or TAT – tired all the time. Research now shows that nearly 80 per cent of people complaining of TAT do get adequate sleep, and that the problem lies in nutritional deficiencies (many sufferers have little interest in food, or eat on the run) which can be cleared up by improving the diet and taking a good multi-vitamin and mineral supplement.

INSOMNIA

Insomnia is considered to be a 'primary sleep disorder', in which you find it difficult to fall asleep, and then sleep only for short periods. There are many causes of insomnia, and fortunately almost all can be treated. Most of us will suffer from insomnia at some point in our lives, from one of the following causes:

- The main cause of insomnia is stress or worry; waking in the middle of the night or very early, and being unable to get back to sleep, is a common characteristic of insomnia, which, unfortunately, also becomes more frequent with age.
- Caffeine is a common cause of insomnia, as is alcohol, which may send you off to sleep, but which has a short-lived effect.
- Pain and depression are common causes.
- Pregnancy and menopausal symptoms may cause insomnia in some women.
- Spinal problems, especially at the top of the spine, can affect sleep.

Other causes include: food allergies, nutritional deficiencies, thyroid disorders, being overtired (you need energy to sleep and to be able to relax), lack of fresh air and exercise, chronic problems such as skin rashes, digestive disorders, asthma and catarrh, and acute problems such as infections, toothaches, earaches, coughs, colds, fever and headaches.

PRACTICAL HELP FOR SLEEP PROBLEMS

- Eat a variety of foods, with plenty of fresh fruit and vegetables. If your sleep problem or fatigue is linked to poor nutrition, this should help to iron it out.
- Avoid sugars, chocolate, cola drinks, nicotine, tea and coffee, all of which have toxins that can affect the nervous system and prevent sleep.
- Avoid eating just before bedtime.
- Avoid excess alcohol, which may act as a depressant in small quantities, but which stimulates the system when you drink too much. You may pass out, but you won't sleep well!
- Eat plenty of food containing calcium, which may encourage sleep. Foods rich in calcium include: parsley, dairy produce, broccoli, dried figs and sesame seeds.
- Take a zinc supplement just before bedtime.
- The amino acid tryptophan helps to encourage healthy sleep – good sources include avocados, turkey, bananas or peanut butter.
- Stop working at least an hour before bedtime, and try reading something light.
- Take more exercise, preferably earlier in the day.
- Take a warm (not hot) bath each night before bed, which will serve the dual purpose of relaxing you and also subconsciously 'washing away' the problems of the day.
- If you cannot get to sleep, switch on the light and read, or do something different, and then try again.
- If you are over-tired when you go to bed, try taking a short afternoon nap, to break the cycle.
- Remove the clock from your bedroom.
- Make an early start. If you want to sleep at night, get up early in the morning, every morning including week-ends. Regularity is important in keeping body rhythms constant.
- Get active. If you don't get enough exercise, your body will be physically underused, causing disturbed or restless sleep. Sleep is a

natural response to physical tiredness, and by increasing your intake of regular exercise, you are likely to increase your amount of deep sleep.

- Create a sanctuary. Take a good look at your bedroom and ask yourself if it is really a place of rest, relaxation and intimacy. Bedrooms are not for work or worry and if your bedroom serves as an office or the household filing cabinet, it's time to make changes.

NATURAL REMEDIES TO HELP YOU SLEEP

There are a host of complementary, natural treatments which will prevent the need for sleeping drugs – the most common medication prescribed today. Some of the following remedies may help you to sleep, and to establish a healthy sleeping pattern:

HOMEOPATHY

Remedies can be taken an hour before going to bed, for up to 14 days. Repeat the dose if you wake in the night, and cannot get back to sleep. Insomnia is usually treated 'constitutionally', which means a remedy is specifically tailored to your individual needs, so you may need to consult a registered homeopath for treatment. The following may be helpful:

- Coffea, when your mind is overactive, and you are unable to switch off.
- Niax, when your sleeplessness is exacerbated by food or alcohol: you wake at around 3 or 4am, then fall asleep just as it is time to get up and are irritable during the day.
- Pulsatilla, when you are restless in the early hours of sleep, feeling uncomfortable, hot and then cold, not thirsty and sleeping with the arms above the head.
- Arnica, when the bed feels too hard, and you are overtired, fidgety and dream of being chased by animals.
- Lycopodium, when your mind is active at bedtime, going over and over work done that day. You dream a lot, talk and laugh in your sleep, and wake at around 4am.
- Arsenicum, when you wake between midnight and 2am, restless, worried and apprehensive.

- Rhus tox, when you cannot sleep, are irritable, restless and feel a need to walk about. Especially useful if there is pain.
- Aurum, when you have dreams about dying, hunger, or problems at work, and become depressed.
- Aconite, when sleep problems are worse after shock. There is restlessness, nightmares and fear of dying.
- Chamomilla, when you are feeling irritable at the beginning of the night, and are unable to sleep. You may want comfort.

HERBAL REMEDIES

- A warm bath with an infusion (herbs steeped in boiling water) of chamomile or lavender will help to relax you.
- A cup of warm herb tea just before bed will soothe and help you to relax. Try chamomile, catnip, lemon balm and limeflowers.
- Make a lavender cushion with dried lavender flowers or seeds, and place it under your pillow.
- A hot footbath before bed helps relaxation by drawing blood away from the head; add a little mustard powder to the water to increase the effect.

AROMATHERAPY

- A few drops of chamomile oil, clary sage or lavender can be added to the bath to relax and encourage sleep.
- Try a gentle massage just before bedtime, with a few drops of chamomile, lavender, rose or neroli in a light carrier oil, such as grapeseed.
- Place a few drops of lavender oil on your bedroom lightbulb just before bed, or place a few drops on a handkerchief and tie it to the bed.

BACH FLOWER REMEDIES

Worrying thoughts and mental arguments might respond to white chestnut; indecision can be treated with scleranthus; stress, strain, frustration and inability to relax respond to vervain, rock water, vine, elm, beech or impatiens. There are many other remedies. Bach flower essences are sold in most good chemists and health shops.

4. Here's looking at you...

YOU ARE ALMOST certain to look better when you feel good, and the reverse also holds true. Dressing in clothes that make you feel comfortable and attractive, holding yourself properly and exuding a positive self-image, can all have a dramatic effect on both your self-esteem and your overall appearance.

However, confidence and self-esteem aren't matters of age or appearance, but of attitude. A confident, self-assured person looks, feels and carries themselves like they are young, fit and attractive. A self-assured person is also more likely to respect his or her body by eating well, getting exercise and avoiding harmful traps like overeating, drinking too much alcohol and taking drugs. It's all part of the same parcel – if you like yourself, you'll treat yourself well. You'll feel better and you'll hold yourself with confidence. You will probably be inspired to dress in clothes that compound that feeling, and to adopt a positive approach to life. That's what this chapter is all about – feeling good about yourself and looking great to boot.

You don't need to be thin to achieve wonderful things, nor do you need to spend a lot of money on clothes. One of the secrets of looking good is to buy clothes that suit your colouring, your mood and your body shape. There are also lots of tricks that can help you feel better about yourself, and hide the things that bother you about your body.

A POSITIVE SELF-IMAGE

Let's start on the inside and work out. You want to give an impression that you are in control,

that you like who you are, that you are self-confident and interesting. Even if you are normally a shrinking violet, it's perfectly possible to change the way you look and the way people perceive you by sending out positive messages.

To attain a positive self-image you have to start by changing your attitude. Attitudes are crucially important to happiness because they define the way we react to the world. They can make the difference between pain and pleasure, misery and happiness and even good and bad health. Your attitude to the world around you involves choices: you can see things positively, or you can see things negatively. Be positive and you allow a little ray of sunshine into your mind and your heart.

Paula Tilbrook
✿ *Always wear what you feel comfortable in, then you are more likely to feel confident and happy with yourself. I enjoy wearing flowing theatrical clothes that are bold in colour – a far cry from Betty's rubber gloves.*

Many people think that feeling good is just something that happens when we feel happy – it's a great feeling and it's nice when it occurs. But research shows that it is an absolute necessity for good health and a long life. Feelings of pleasure and well-being are signals of satisfaction from the same part of the brain that controls important body functions, such as your immune and cardiovascular systems. When you are unhappy, when your well-being is at a low ebb, your other systems are compromised and your defences are weakened. So not only is a good, positive attitude important for feeling good, it's also crucial to health.

Here's how to begin:

■ Look at things positively. If things go wrong,

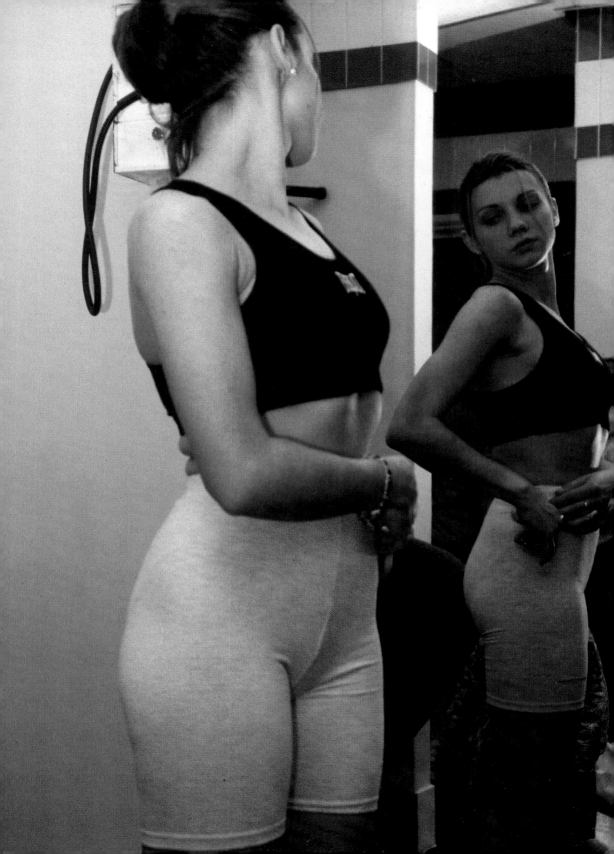

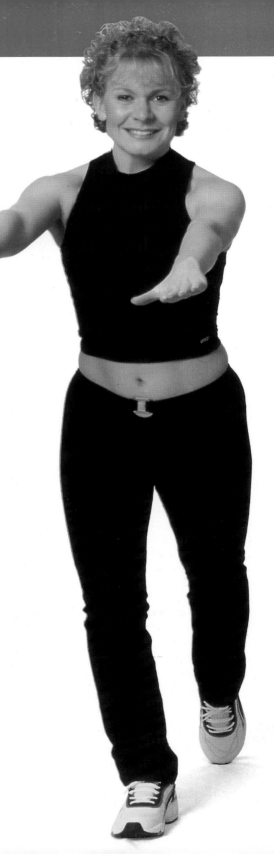

stop and consider the worst possible
scenario. Once you've come to grips with
that, you'll be prepared for whatever comes
your way and, with a little advance planning,
you'll be equipped to cope.

- Practise some positive affirmations (see page
  57). Start with phrases, such as: I am
  confident, I am happy, I am a person other
  people would like to get to know, I am
  popular, I like myself. It might sound
  silly, but keep it up. Eventually
  these phrases will become
  embedded in your
  subconscious and you'll
  really believe them. Make your
  affirmations a self-fulfilling prophecy.
- Smile. Even if you are feeling low, try to
  summon up a smile. It's well known that
  smiling releases the 'happy' chemicals of the
  brain, so even if you have to work hard to
  smile, you'll be part-way to feeling better.
  Smiling also encourages other people to
  smile back – which can't help but make you
  feel good. There is no question that people
  are more attracted to a smiling, happy
  person than a person who looks miserable.
- Stand up straight and pull your shoulders
  back (see page 58). You'll look more
  confident and you'll probably feel it too.
- Chat. Small talk might not be your strong
  point, but if you stop and talk to people, and
  show interest in them, you'll appear more
  interesting and approachable. If you're stuck
  for a topic, you can always discuss the
  weather.
- Stride out. Put a spring in your step. Activity
  gets your blood moving, taking oxygen to
  your brain and all the other important parts
  of your body. You'll also look happy and
  confident – a sure-fire way to success.
- Dress the part. Dress in colours that you
  find uplifting. Choose clothes that make you
  feel good (see page 64). If you are confident
  about the way you look, other people will
  stop and take note – and you'll feel even
  better.
- Think of the times when people have
  complimented you – maybe asked if you've
  lost weight, or commented on what you were

wearing. On some occasions you may have made no changes at all – you may have been in a good mood, or feeling happy about something. Feeling good changes the way you look and appear to other people. Take advantage of that.

- Savour your successes. We are trained to be modest, but there is no need to belittle your own triumphs. Say to yourself: I worked very hard, I did a good job and I'm proud of myself. That's the optimistic way of thinking about good events that you brought about through your own efforts.
- Make the best of hard times. When you are optimistic, you can believe you can make the most of what you've got. Sometimes you need to redefine your objectives and let go of some expectations. Then just do your best and take pride in little successes.
- Let go of negative thoughts. When you become aware of negative thoughts, you can learn to stop pessimistic thinking. Pinch yourself, or snap an elastic band around your wrist when you find that your optimism is sinking. These techniques may seem drastic, but they can stop a bout of pessimism before it starts.
- My motto is 'you have to go down into the valleys to get up the other side to enjoy the views'. Like everyone else, I have been through hard times, but these days I realise that things will get better and I appreciate and enjoy life all the more for having been through the hard times. I will also have learnt from my tricky periods not to let myself get into that predicament again. THINK POSITIVELY – things can only get better.
- Help others. If things are getting you down, do what you can to help others. Whether you do some volunteer work, make cakes for your children's fête, or just listen to the problems of a friend, you'll be giving, and there's a real sense of fulfilment in that.

When you are appreciated, your spirits are lifted and you feel good about yourself.

BUILDING SELF-CONFIDENCE AND SELF-ESTEEM

It is possible to build self-confidence, even if you have lacked confidence since childhood. Essentially there are four things to remember:

- Confidence is not just one thing. Each of us lacks confidence in some areas of our life, and has confidence in others.
- Apparently confident people around you are not as confident as you think.
- We gain confidence from doing things.
- If you tell people you are no good, they are likely to believe it.

Building self-confidence takes practice. You need to learn to behave as if you are more confident than you feel, and to be flexible in your behaviour. Learn from your mistakes, and understand that mistakes are part of a learning curve. Silence the voice of self-blame and speak encouragingly to yourself. Be kind to yourself.

Having been in the public eye for 11 years, you probably think I should be brimming with confidence, but I always have moments of insecurity, just as I did before I joined *Emmerdale*. When I have doubts in my ability, I talk to myself, assure myself that I can do it: 'Glenda, come on, go for it'. I get really angry with myself sometimes – this tends to work!

To build self-esteem, you need to attack prejudices that led you to undervalue yourself in the first place. Low self-esteem is a prejudice about yourself – seeing yourself as unworthy or unacceptable. The self-perception is biased, or flawed, but you have a hard time seeing it any other way. Learn to acknowledge your qualities rather than discounting them. You also need to learn to

> ➤ **Wear clothes that fit. There's nothing worse than hiking up a pair of too-small tights, or pulling down a pair of too-tight knickers. Tight clothing reminds you that you are, perhaps, heavier than you'd like to be, and it does nothing for your figure. Similarly, if you are thin, hiding beneath a sea. of fabric will not show your body to best advantage and you'll end up looking lost and unsure of yourself.**

stifle your inner critic. Congratulate yourself. See the good in what you have done. Do the best you can, and don't berate yourself for not being perfect. Finally, spend time with people who make you feel good about yourself.

Seek out pleasure and treats. The more you are enjoying yourself, the more relaxed you will feel. Learn to give yourself breaks. Take short breaks, like half an hour talking to a friend, as well as long ones, like regular holidays.

How the mind and body work together is a question to which no one has found a complete answer, but one thing is clear: the mind affects the body and the body affects the mind. In order to keep fit mentally, therefore, you need to attend to your body. That means overcoming problems that affect your body, such as difficulties with sleeping, eating, drinking, smoking, or relying on tranquillizers. Many of these problems involve bad habits. In order to defeat them, you need to make a positive decision to change. Study the habit until you are aware of exactly what you do. Develop a personal strategy for stopping and find something else to do instead. Once you have started, keep the momentum going. Be prepared for setbacks, and remember that the changes you are planning to make are for you. Remind yourself constantly of the reasons why you want to make changes, and visualize the outcome you hope for. This positive reinforcement will help you to succeed.

For example, if you are making changes that involve eating better, taking more exercise and cutting down on bad habits such as smoking or drinking, consider your aims. If you suffer from niggling health problems, such as headaches, lethargy or irritability, imagine yourself being free from these. If you are overweight and want to look and feel better, visualize yourself the way

➤ **Criticism or misunderstood statements from others can create a false image of your body. Did your mother always draw attention to what she perceived to be your figure faults? Does your partner complain about your big bottom or non-existent bust? Don't let them get you down, and keep yesterday's memories where they belong. Accept instead the objective opinions of supportive friends you trust. No matter how you feel about your body, you will definltely have some attractive features. Learn to play up the good, and hide the parts you are less sure about.**

you want to look. Making changes involves focusing on the positive, and celebrating each victory along the way.

POSTURE

Changing your figure by improving your posture is actually one of the oldest tricks in the book. Stand in front of a mirror and let it all hang out. Turn sideways and have a look from that angle, too. Now stand up straight, pull your shoulders back and suck in your tummy. What do you notice? You look slimmer, of course, but you also look more confident and self-assured. It is almost impossible to maintain the 'I'm looking at myself in a mirror' posture for longer than you are actually standing in front of the mirror. This is largely because this 'sucking in' posture, though better, is still incorrect – it's unnatural, stiff, and puts strains on your body. Go back to your relaxed stance and start again. Turn sideways on to the mirror and let yourself droop. Release all the muscles in your abdomen and let your stomach protrude as far as it wants. Collapse your spine and drop your shoulders. Now try the Pilates way to improving your posture correctly.

PILATES FOR POSTURE

Apart from affecting breathing, posture problems give rise directly to specific figure problems. Pilates offers exercises for postural improvements that will open up your chest and help to get some oxygen into your lungs. This has the knock-on effect of energizing your mind and body so you feel great. Here's how to do it:

1. Open your shoulders by allowing your shoulder blades to slide smoothly towards each other across your back and then pull them downwards slightly. Use the muscles in your back to do this rather than forcing with your neck and shoulders.

2. As your shoulders settle into the right position you will feel your neck naturally moving back slightly, allowing your head to come into a direct

balance over the top of the spine.

3. Settle comfortably in this position with your chin and eyes parallel with the ground.

4. Press your feet into the floor, your head to the ceiling and see yourself as a taller person. Imagine you have pockets of air between your vertebrae.

5. Walk with your toes facing forward, chest open and weight of the head directly over the spine.

6. When carrying bags, carry them evenly in both hands, keeping your arms in line with your body.

Sheree Murphy
❀ *I tend to wear clothes which show off the top half of my body, as I don't like drawing attention to my hips and bum. I wear something a bit more daring and colourful on top and I feel more confident like this.*

It is important for your posture to be good before you start the following exercise to improve your breathing, otherwise it will be impossible to move the muscles enough to do the exercise. For the basic Pilates breathing exercise you need a long towel, exercise band or dressing-gown cord. Sit on the edge of a chair with knees hip-width apart and feet flat on the ground. Fold your towel into a long, narrow shape and pass it round your back just below bust level as though you are about to dry your back. At the front, cross the ends over and hold each end tightly so that the towel is firmly wrapped round your rib cage just below your bust line. Now try to take an ordinary breath in

and out. If you are breathing properly you should find that you are unable to do this because the towel is preventing your ribs from moving. Those who breathe shallowly, without using their rib cage, will not find their breathing inhibited.

Now take another, deeper breath in. This time as you breathe in, let the towel move to accommodate your rib movement. Be conscious of your ribs flaring upwards and outwards to make space for the maximum amount of air to come into your lungs. Be aware of how much the towel has to give to allow for this expansion. When you breathe out, don't let the air come gusting out anyhow. Try to use your muscles to push it out properly from the bottom, as if squeezing toothpaste out of a tube. Notice how much looser the towel is when you have finished breathing out. Once you have practised this technique using the towel, put it into action in your day to day life.

Improved posture has many benefits. Standing up straight can improve your metabolism to help achieve fat loss. There are other improvements throughout the system, including better digestion and health, less fatigue and a general sense of enhanced well-being and self-esteem.

THE ALEXANDER TECHNIQUE

The Alexander Technique is a process of re-education which aims to teach us to rediscover our natural poise and balance, and use our bodies more efficiently. It is often referred to as 'posture training', but this term touches on only one element of the theory behind the technique.

The Alexander Technique is taught in lessons where the practitioner is referred to as a 'teacher' and the individual taking the lessons is known as a 'pupil'. The lessons focus on improving physical and psychological well-being by reducing muscular tension and encouraging a more poised and integrated use of the body. It is now recognized as one of the most important

➤ **Men, just like women, admire an enormous range of physical types. There are men who go for only thin women, men who go for only very large women and men who will go for any body type, provided they like the woman's looks, conversation, intelligence, humour and all the rest. The trouble is, we don't always believe that we are loveable. When boyfriends claim to like our curvaceous thighs, we think they are mad or lying. Learn to accept yourself – and to accept that you are loveable and attractive to someone else. You'll appear a lot more attractive if you feel good and give off a positive vibe. We all know people who have serious figure flaws and attract the opposite sex like bees to honey. What do they have? Confidence! Confidence is sexy. If you believe you look great, others will believe it too!**

SO WHAT SHAPE ARE YOU?

Coming to terms with your body shape can be liberating. You can throw away those too-tight jeans and slide into something that draws attention to your curvy hips. You can give up on the long skirts you thought made you look tall and willowy, and try a pair of pedal-pushers instead. Short, tall, slim, curvy or bordering on the far side of plump, there are clothes to suit you, and once you've accepted that the figure you've got is yours come feast or famine, you can take positive steps to settle on a look that you like and, most importantly, feel comfortable in. You can start to look better immediately by dressing for what you are, rather than what you would like to be.

Janet Menzies, author of *Cheat at Slimming* (Hodder & Stoughton), has come up with a brilliant analysis of body types, which is adapted here. In her book, she explains that body type is determined by genetics and can be changed only very little. There are three main body types: endomorphic (rounded); mesomorphic (muscular); and ectomorphic (lanky). All three types have good and bad points. Mesomorphs for example, often look better undressed than dressed, whereas ectomorphs are the opposite.

Go through the questions and statements below, honestly noting which is most accurate for you, then check to discover your body type and figure shape.

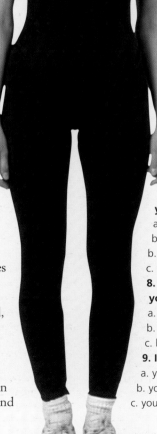

1. Is your height:
a. below average?
b. average?
c. above average?

2. Is your face shape:
a. round?
b. square or heart-shape?
c. oval or oblong?

3. Are your feet and hands:
a. small and plump?
b. average size but broad?
c. long and narrow?

4. Are your arms and legs:
a. short and rounded in appearance?
b. average size, chunky looking?
c. long and slender?

5. Which of the following statements describes you most closely?
a. small and chubby
b. stocky, muscular
c. tall and willowy

6. With which of these problems do you identify most?
a. I gain weight very easily
b. I find exercise more helpful than dieting but I always seem to look muscular
c. I've always been skinny

7. When buying clothes, which is your biggest problem?
a. skirts too small, jackets too large when buying suits
b. tops too small
c. waist too tight, hips too baggy

8. Which object would you compare yourself with?
a. apple or pear
b. hourglass
c. banana

9. Is your best feature:
a. your bust and shoulders?
b. your waist?
c. your legs?

ANSWERS

Mostly As – Endomorph (rounded)

If you scored mostly As on the questionnaire, then your body type is that of a typical endomorph. You probably don't need telling that this body type could be summed up in one word: rounded. The classic endomorph has lots of round shapes in her body. Her face tends to be round and she usually has a thicker layer of subcutaneous fat which gives her arms, legs and torso a rounded appearance. Endomorphs are usually shorter than average height, and their small (often round-looking) feet and hands are a tell-tale pointer to their body type.

Endomorphs are more prone to fat than other body types and have to work harder to stay slim than ectomorphs do. But if you are an endomorph at least you can take comfort from the knowledge that in this country at least, you are not alone. Laying down extra fat, and putting it on round the lower half of the body are also feminine traits, dictated by female hormones. So endomorphic qualifies are really very natural and normal for any woman – but unfortunately being the norm doesn't make them fashionable. Every endomorph is all too aware that hers is not the shape of the moment, while her exact opposite, the tall, slim willowy ectomorph is.

Mostly Bs – Mesomorph (muscular)

The mesomorph – literally 'middle shape' – body type is in fact less common than its name suggests. Its chief characteristic is muscularity, and since women are less muscular than men, the mesomorphic build tends to be more common among men. Mesomorphs are usually of average height, with a square or heart-shaped face. The mesomorphic build gives an appearance of strength – and is often athletic and strong. The skeleton of a mesomorph tends to be broader, with stronger, thicker individual bones than either the endomorph or the ectomorph. A classic give-away of a big-boned, mesomorphic structure is thick wrists and broad hands and feet. If a mesomorph is fit, their bones are the frame for large, efficient muscles capable of explosive action like sprinting. If the mesomorph is unfit, she is prone to laying down fat instead of muscle. Either way, the general appearance can look chunky and stocky.

This rather dense build is the down-side of being mesomorphic. Madonna made a typical mesomorphic transition from slightly plump and chunky at the beginning of her career to lean and muscular after she started working out, but she still isn't willowy, and never will be. The plus side of this is that the mesomorphic build is the most easily sculpted to create the body-shape you want. You can't change the shape of bones or fat, but you can alter the size, length and bulk of muscles, and since mesomorphs are more muscular, their bodies respond well to the use of weights, or yoga and pilates.

I am mesomorphic and to be honest I would hate to be too willowy and tall to get stuck into sport. I always used to wish I was slimmer and taller but you have to learn to live with and love what you have. My body is short and muscular but it is firm, toned and shapely – I can live with that!

True mesomorphs also find physical exercise easier than the rest of us and therefore usually positively enjoy it, though endomorphs will find this hard to believe. So if you are mesomorphic, it's time to stop bemoaning your stockiness and start to make your body type work for you. A bonus is that the two most common mesomorphic figure shapes are currently rather fashionable (indeed they are rarely out of favour with men).

Mostly Cs – Ectomorph (rangy)

If you have scored mostly Cs, prepare to be an object of envy, because you have the current 'in' shape, the ectomorph. You are above average height, with long legs and slender arms. You actually find it hard to gain fat and stay naturally willowy most of the time – and we all hate you. Ectomorphs rapidly become used to this lack of sympathy from their non-ectomorph friends, but in fact there are down-sides to this body type just as there are with the other two. Many ectomorphs would love to have curves: they hated being called bean-poles at school and long for a bust and a peach-shaped bottom.

Lack of strength and a difficulty In maintaining any sort of figure can also be a problem for ectomorphs. Throughout most of northern Europe the ectomorphic build is fairly rare for women, so many ectomorphs become self-conscious about the fact that they almost literally stick out at social gatherings. Many end up modelling just to be among similar-looking people to themselves, and most fashion models today are ectomorphs. Hard as it is for non-ectomorphs to believe, ectomorphs can have figure problems.

In her book, *Cheat at Slimming*, Janet Menzies offers ways to hide the features you hate, while accentuating those that make you feel good. She also offers exercise tips to blitz problem areas. It's a book well worth investing in!

REMEDIES FOR A POSITIVE APPROACH TO LIFE

It's not easy to have a positive attitude when you are feeling down in the dumps. All of us have periods when life seems more difficult, and it's perfectly acceptable to get some help with our outlook.

Possibly the best remedies for negative emotions are the Bach flower remedies, which work to balance negative or unhappy feelings so that you feel yourself again. They can also help to overcome lifelong patterns of behaviour or emotions that have been difficult to shift. If you find it difficult to face a crowded room, you feel depressed about your body or you feel sluggish and lacking in enthusiasm, it's possible to change your outlook using these remedies. There are 38 Bach flower remedies, all of which address the whole spectrum of negative emotions. Here are some of the ones that might be most appropriate:

Agrimony
For those who hide their feelings behind a cheerful face. They claim that all is well even when it is not.

Beech
For the perfectionist who finds it hard to tolerate or understand the shortcomings of those they believe to be foolish, short-sighted or ignorant.

Centaury
For those who are kind, gentle and eager to please, but so unwilling to let anyone down that they find it impossible to say no.

Elm
For those who are overwhelmed and made to feel inadequate by pressure from work, family and other commitments.

Gentian
For the eternal pessimist who is easily discouraged. Even when they are doing well, small setbacks dishearten them.

Gorse
For those who believe that they were born to suffer and are pessimistic about everything.

Holly
For those who develop the victim mentality and are overcome with hatred, jealousy, envy or suspicion. They may keep their feelings to themselves, but burn with resentment against others.

and useful methods of maintaining health and encouraging the efficiency of our bodies.

The Alexander Technique will help you to:
- become aware of yourself on a holistic level – mind, body and spirit;
- prevent unnecessary strain on your body;
- use energy more efficiently, preventing fatigue;
- rediscover the grace you had as a child.

STANDING
Most of us stand in ways that put enormous strain on our bodies. Observe yourself in the mirror and objectively analyse the ways in which you could improve your posture. Unbalanced posture can put strain on your entire skeletal system and internal organs, so it is important that you address your posture as soon as possible.

Stand in front of the mirror as you would normally, and make sure you feel comfortable. Ask yourself the following questions:
- Is my weight equally balanced or am I standing more on one leg than the other? Move back and forth to find a position that feels right for you, and you'll soon notice if one leg feels more comfortable with the bulk

Impatiens
For those who do everything in a hurry. They are brusque, finish sentences for people, fidget, look at their watch and edge towards the door while others are still talking. The remedy encourages calm, tolerance and patience.

Larch
For those with ability but no confidence. They need to believe in themselves and not miss opportunities because of self doubt and feelings of inferiority.

Mimulus
For those who are shy, nervous and blush easily. They feel uneasy with people they do not know, dislike parties and feel self-conscious.

Mustard
For those who are gloomy for no apparent reason. The mood can sometimes stay months before it goes.

Olive
For those who are exhausted due to overwork or over-exertion, when they have no energy or strength left and life is no longer fun.

Walnut
This is the remedy for change. It settles a person into a new environment and helps them cope with life changes such as marriage, divorce, birth, puberty, the menopause.

Water Violet
For the reserved, self contained and dignified. They like peace and quiet, but can seem aloof and their need for privacy may lead them to become isolated.

Wild oat
For those who are dithering at a cross-roads in life. They are discontented with their career or lifestyle and

may want something more fulfilling, but do not know where to look.

Wild rose
For those who drift and have neither the enthusiasm nor ambition to change any aspect of their life. They let illness and misfortune triumph over them and are willing to accept whatever fate delivers.

Willow
For the grouchy, introspective pessimist, who dwells on misfortune and wallows in self-pity. They feel that life has dealt them a poor hand and cannot think what they have done to deserve it. They sulk when things go wrong.

of the weight than the other.

■ Do I stand on the inside or outside of my feet, or is my weight firmly placed on the centre of my feet? Don't be surprised if each foot is different. You may stand on the inside of one, and on the outside of the other, depending on which leg carries the most weight.

■ Do I lean forward or back? In other words, is most of the weight on the front of your feet (the balls) or on your heels?
■ Are my knees locked or relaxed? Do you feel most comfortable with them bent (which may indicate that they are over-relaxed) or are they firm?

Look at your shoes to see where you tend to put the most weight. They will be worn down in places where there is more pressure.

Move back and forth and reassume your position. When you think you have noticed habits indicating misuse, such as putting more weight on one leg than the other,

Malandra Burrows
✿ *I always choose clothes which reflect my mood that day. This means I always feel comfortable, even when it is a black day!*

exaggerate that stance. This will give you an idea of the tensions that this position creates in your body. Exaggerate every stance that seems incorrect, and you will begin to understand better how your body works both in and out of balance.

There is not one correct way of standing, but the Alexander Technique provides a list of useful suggestions to bear in mind while we do so.

- The feet could be at a 45-degree angle, with about 9 inches (23 cm) between them. This provides a solid base on which the body can be supported.
- When standing for long periods of time, place one foot slightly behind the other, with the weight of the body resting mainly on the rear foot. This will help you to avoid shifting your weight from one hip to another, which is a primary cause of posture imbalance.
- Allow your hips to shift back as far as is comfortable, without affecting your balance or throwing your body forward. Many of us shift our pelvises forward when we stand, and this exercise will help to prevent that tendency.
- There are three points on the foot which form a triangle upon which we should rest our weight. Using all three gives us the best possible base upon which to balance, and we will avoid overusing muscles in an attempt to keep upright. The three points which form the triangle are the heel, the ball of the foot below the big toe, and the base of the little toe.

Studies show that both anxiety and depression respond to the Alexander Technique, by reducing the effects of stress on the body, and by improving overall body image. A better body image and an enhanced sense of well-being will also allow you to become calmer and more

Freya Copeland
✿ I always wear black when I want to look tall and slim. Black definitely has a slimming effect.
✿ Back at school when I was a lot heavier, one of the girls I used to admire for style told me: never wear more than three colours at once. I always follow this rule as it keep things stylish and uncomplicated, and is much more flattering to the figure.
✿ I always wear hipster trousers as I feel they are a lot more flattering than trousers that split you in two round your waist.

capable of dealing with problems.

WHAT'S YOUR SHAPE?

You might aspire to the Kate Moss look, but if you've got hips that bring to mind Rubens rather than Vogue, you're unlikely to manage it. Maybe you long for Marilyn Monroe-esque curves, when your bust is firmly situated in the A-section of the lingerie department. The secret to looking good is a little self-awareness. There are lots of ways to make yourself look fabulous, whatever your shape. But you have to know and accept your shape before you can perform any wardrobe wonders. There is no point in going for a look that your shape will never suit. Instead, find a look that accentuates your figure and focuses on its very best features.

CHOOSING THE RIGHT CLOTHES

If thighs are your problem:

- Avoid wearing clothes that are too tight, unless your curves can sustain them.
- Choose skirts and dresses that sit just below the narrowest part of your leg (just above the knee, or at the ankle). Mid-knee length is normally good. If you want to go mini, choose a short A-line skirt that flares slightly from the hips.
- Wear high heels to lengthen your legs and give an illusion of height.
- Choose trousers that widen gradually from the hipbones. Flares and bootleg trousers draw attention downwards away from the hips and thighs.
- Choose sheer, control-top or contour tights.

BIG BOTTOMS

- Enhance the top half of your body to provide balance – go for hour-glass, rather than trying to hide your bottom half.
- Choose skirts that drape rather than cling.

- Avoid pleats and heavily gathered waistlines.
- Concentrate on clothes that fit the hips and legs rather than the waist. A loose waistband is a lesser evil than a skirt or pair of trousers that hug your hips, bulges and all.
- Wear big sweaters and shirts, that end just below the hips. Choose A-line or straight tops that fall directly from the shoulders.
- Try to keep the bottom and top halves of your body in the same or similar colours to avoid sharp contrasts that draw the eye to the part you want to hide.
- Choose slim-fitting trousers with a side zip and no pockets to draw attention to problem areas.

FLABBY TUMMIES

- Wear a belt to define the waist area, creating an hour-glass rather than a ripe apple look.
- Avoid pockets or details on the abdominal area. Clean, straight lines are best.
- Try dresses that fall from the bust. If you are shapely up on top, they'll draw attention to one of your best features and hide that flabby tummy.
- Avoid tight skirts or trousers that stretch across your belly.
- Avoid heavy pleats that will sit uncomfortably.
- Try A-line skirts without a centre-front zip.
- Neat, straight trousers without front pockets or front zips will also help to give a nice silhouette.
- Loose T-shirts and sweaters over slim-leg trousers will give a longer, leaner look.

BUSTING OUT

- Avoid fussy necklines or patterns that draw attention upwards. Sleek polo necks are good, as are V-neck tops that draw the eye downward.
- Avoid pleats and gathers in the chest area, concentrating instead on slimming, long lines.
- Fitted tops are better than very loose ones, which may give the appearance that the rest of your body is as big as your bust.
- Get a well-fitting bra that lifts and defines. Your bust can be your asset, so don't be tempted to hunch your shoulders and hide it.
- Avoid dresses and shirts with a low bustline or too-narrow straps.

FEELING SHORT-CHANGED?

- Try a padded bra, or a good bra that makes the most of what you have.
- Don't hesitate to wear tight tops that accentuate your bust. Detail across the bustline is ideal for focusing on the curves you do have.

HEAVILY ARMED

- Show as much shoulder as you can, if you are choosing sleeveless tops. It's best to see the whole arm rather than cutting it in half, or creating a line at the widest part.
- Choose a sleeve length that ends at the narrowest part of your arm.
- Avoid tight armholes or anything that cuts into the flesh of your arm.
- Try fitted, three-quarter length sleeves that draw attention to the slimmer forearm.

Alyson Spiro

✿ *I dress to suit my figure, I never wear anything too tight around my middle – I don't want to draw attention to that area as I have carried three children.*

✿ *I believe that dressing to express yourself makes you feel good about yourself. I like wearing real one-offs. I wore a very colourful sari to the 'Soap Awards' this year, and it made me feel very much in control and confident in myself.*

This chapter can help you to an extent but you really have to help yourself – believe me, I've been there, like every single person reading this book. I've told myself over and over again, 'You aren't as fat as you think you are, you aren't as ugly as you think you are,' and it's worked! A positive body image has helped me leave my childhood bout of anorexia well in the past and I've moved on to feeling more confident, which naturally translates into looking more confident and feeling great.

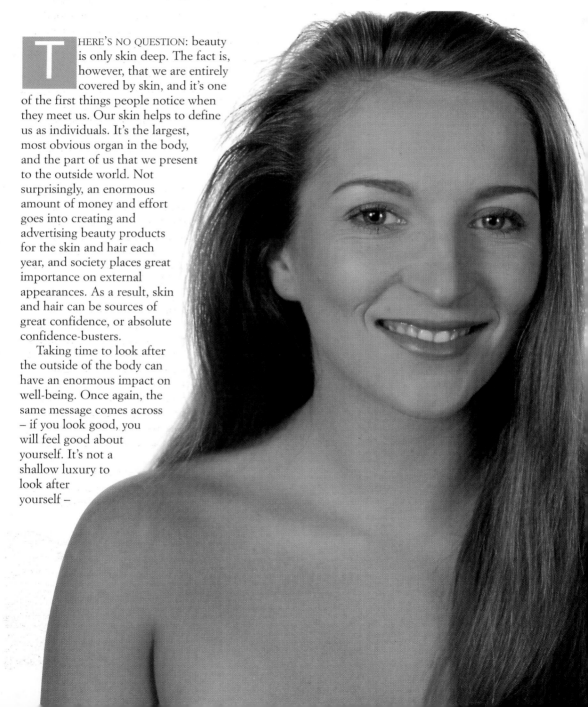

5. Body beautiful

THERE'S NO QUESTION: beauty is only skin deep. The fact is, however, that we are entirely covered by skin, and it's one of the first things people notice when they meet us. Our skin helps to define us as individuals. It's the largest, most obvious organ in the body, and the part of us that we present to the outside world. Not surprisingly, an enormous amount of money and effort goes into creating and advertising beauty products for the skin and hair each year, and society places great importance on external appearances. As a result, skin and hair can be sources of great confidence, or absolute confidence-busters.

Taking time to look after the outside of the body can have an enormous impact on well-being. Once again, the same message comes across – if you look good, you will feel good about yourself. It's not a shallow luxury to look after yourself –

it's one of the keys to positive emotional health. Obviously changes to diet, exercise and stress levels will have a dramatic effect on the health of skin and hair – and overall appearance – but there are many tricks of the trade that can help you look great from head to toe, with the minimum of fuss.

SKINCARE

Safeguarding your skin doesn't have to take much time at all. And despite all the advertising hype that surrounds the big name brands and unbelievably time-consuming beauty routines, it doesn't have to be complicated or expensive.

WHY YOU NEED TO LOOK AFTER YOUR SKIN

As well as providing the body with protection, your skin is the interface between the body's internal structures and the environment, playing a vital role in temperature regulation, sensory perception and some immune responses. It has the dual ability of absorbing some things and excreting others. Be very careful what you put on your skin because it readily absorbs substances, which then pass into the blood stream to be transported around the whole body. Similarly, you can help the skin in its excretory functions by keeping it clean, allowing it to 'breathe' by wearing natural fibres, and by not using substances such as anti-perspirants, which make its job more difficult.

To see how efficiently the skin absorbs and transports substances around the body, try this: rub a clove of fresh garlic on the skin of your foot. Within five minutes, you'll smell it on your breath. This exercise should certainly make the majority of us think carefully about what it is we are applying to our skin, either to nourish and protect it, or to treat common ailments.

PAULA TILBROOK
❀ *I have dry skin and recommend washing your face only once every twenty-four hours with soap and water, otherwise you will dry the skin out even more.*
❀ *As an older woman, I would say that, as far as make-up is concerned, less is more.*

THE INSIDE OUT

Maintaining healthy skin starts with a good diet. This means a varied diet with plenty of fresh fruit and vegetables, and lots of whole grains. Avoid too much fatty, greasy or refined foods and additives. Too much alcohol and smoking has a very detrimental effect on the skin.

Clean, fresh air is absolutely necessary for healthy skin, and this can be problematic for anyone living in a city or by a busy road. Regular cleansing is important to clear your pores of dirt.

Apply a good plant-based moisturizer regularly to help protect and nourish the skin.

WRINKLES

Doctors say that the inevitable wrinkles from genetics and gravity shouldn't arrive until you are near your sixties. But they come a lot earlier – in the twenties and thirties for many of us. Here's why.

During the 1920s, French designer Coco Chanel came back from the tropics bronzed and glowing, and the centuries-old tradition of keeping skin in the shade was lost. Fashion conscious women everywhere began to bask in the sun. They started a new trend of sunburn and tanning booths, and skin cancer and early wrinkles. Even in naturally dark skin, sun damage causes 80 to 90 per cent of the visible signs of ageing.

The number two cause of wrinkles is smoking, which speeds up your skin's ageing by up to ten years. Smoking reduces blood flow to the skin, blunting its ability to repair damage. It also sets off enzymes that attack the tissues of your skin. And because skin develops a 'memory' when it is folded in the same place over and over again, the

> ➤ Hop in the bath while the water is still running, and then add a little coconut oil to the hot water tap. The 'oil' will melt into the water and leave your skin wonderfully soft.

mechanics of smoking cause wrinkles too.

Some lines will form simply because we express emotion, with a ready smile or worried frown. The way you sleep can leave a wrinkle memory in your skin, too, especially if you sleep face down.

WHAT CAN YOU DO?

- Sunscreen is the best weapon against further sun damage. Use a full spectrum sunscreen on your face that blocks out both kinds of ultraviolet radiation (UVA and UVB), and use it every day, all year round.
- Read your sunscreen package. The best of the broad-spectrum sunscreens contain titanium dioxide, which stays in your skin and resists washing off.
- To moisturize dry skin, use pure olive oil and calendula cream. Apply them sparingly to the face.
- Excessive washing tends to dry the skin, but skin brushing, with a dry loofah or soft brush, is very beneficial because it removes dead cells from the epidermis (top layers of the skin) and gently massages the blood and lymph vessels in the dermis (lower layers of the skin), speeding up the elimination of toxins.
- Facial gymnastics, systematically exercising the main muscle groups in the face, also help to keep the skin youthful and supple.
- Drink plenty of fresh, plain water, which helps the body to remove toxins more efficiently, and keeps the skin clear, plump and moist. Spritzing it throughout the day will help the top layer to absorb moisture.
- Always put oils in your bath after you've soaked in the tub for a few moments. Oil seals moisture in, but if it's there before your body has had a chance to absorb the water, the oil will seal it out.

SKINCARE TIPS

- Wash your face no more than twice a day. Cleansing too often will only make dry skin drier and oily skin more oily.
- Dilute your cleanser with lots of water when you wash to make it gentler on the skin.
- Using toners with alcohol may feel great, but

Alyson Spiro

❀ *I never bother with fancy packaged, fancy-priced skin-care stuff. I don't even use soap, just plain old-fashioned water and my skin is in really good condition. All those fancy products do is dry out your skin.*

❀ *I have constantly dyed my hair so, to keep it in good condition, I always condition thoroughly.*

they can dry out and irritate the skin. Stick to toners without an alcohol base.
- Too much scrubbing will make your skin flaky. Avoid abrasive facial pads and grainy facial scrubs.
- Facial cleansers can leave an invisible residue behind which can clog your pores. Rinse three times, then rinse again.
- Forget about harsh cleansers and astringents. Inexpensive, mild soaps (such as Dove, or Neutrogena) are all you need to keep your skin clean. If your skin is very dry, you might find that soap exacerbates it. Instead, use gentle creamy cleansing lotions that do not contain soap.
- Keep your water temperature warm, never hot, which can burn the skin. It's a nice idea to splash with cold water afterwards, but it will not 'close your pores', as previously believed.
- Be gentle when you dry your skin. Rubbing with a hard towel can cause tiny abrasions which can gather bacteria and lead to break outs. The idea is to leave a thin film of moisture on your skin, and then to use a moisturizer to trap it.
- If you want to use a toner, try a soothing flower water, such as rose water, after you cleanse and rinse. Toners will temporarily close pores, which is useful before applying make-up, for instance.
- A good everyday moisturizer should be 'noncomedogenic', which means it will not clog your pores. Try to choose products that say noncomedogenic on the label.
- Moisturize around the eyes gently only at night. Don't worry about using expensive

creams or lotions, petroleum jelly or aqueous cream is just as effective as any brand name.

THE MALE REVOLUTION

Skincare is as important for men as it is for women, but only recently have products designed specifically for men become widely available – and acceptable. There's no need to spend a lot of money on skincare products, but most men need more than a splash of aftershave to keep their skin looking fresh and healthy. Here are some tips for keeping skin clean, healthy and youthful.

- Shaving removes the top layer of dead cells that make your skin look dull. It can give you a cleaner, younger appearance, but only if you treat your skin well.
- If you use an electric razor, shave before you shower or wash. The oils that build up on your face overnight will act as a protective barrier between your skin and the razor.
- Prepare your skin with a preshave that does not contain alcohol, which can be drying.
- Before shaving, splash your face with lots of lukewarm water. It will soften hairs and make them easier to cut, no matter what type of razor you use. After you lather on your shaving cream, wait two or three minutes to allow the product to soften the whiskers.
- Don't pull your face tight when you shave. It will eventually cause it to sag and lose its firmness.
- Shave in the direction that your beard grows. If you shave against the grain, you'll cut the whiskers too short, and they will spring back below the surface of the skin. When they begin to grow again, the hair follicles will become inflamed, causing sore little red bumps.
- Aftershaves aren't a great idea – they can irritate and dehydrate the skin. If you are attached to your brand, dilute it with lots of water before applying. A better idea is to splash with cool water, or a little diluted witch hazel.
- Use a gentle soap on your face and don't scrub. Deodorant soaps might be all right for areas of the body that perspire (although they can be drying), but they are not ideal for the face and softer areas, of the body.
- Use lukewarm, never hot water, which can be drying.
- Always use a moisturizer. If you apply it to damp skin, it will help to seal in the moisture. If you hate a greasy feeling, choose a light moisturizer designed for everyday use. Leave it on for at least ten minutes, and then dab it with a towel to remove any excess.
- Use a high protection sunscreen (see page 68), which will prevent sun damage and wrinkles.

Steve Magan

✿ *I don't use any male skin care products. I have tried them and they just dried out my skin really badly. The best thing to do with your skin is not a lot! If you over-interfere with it you will damage it.*

✿ *If I am off work for a few days I let my beard grow. This gives the skin a break from shaving irritation.*

With having to wear a lot of makeup in my job, I treat myself to a trip to the beautician once a month for a deep cleaning facial. I really see the difference when I come out. My skin feels so smooth and looks so clear that I really don't want to put makeup on it again.

WATCH THAT SUN

As the days become longer, and the weather hots up for summer, most of us feel better, happier, less stressed and more optimistic. Naturally, the arrival of the holiday season does much to lift spirits, but there are other factors at work. Sunlight is proven to affect our moods. The pineal gland in the centre of the brain produces melatonin, a chemical that helps to regulate the sleep–wake cycle. We produce melatonin when it's dark, and stop producing it when it's light. If there's too much darkness (and too much melatonin), other brain chemicals are affected – particularly our production of serotonin, the 'feel-good' substance. Interestingly, the anti-depressant drug

Prozac works by raising serotonin levels, so it's not surprising that sunlight, which naturally lifts serotonin levels, also improves mood.

Living in a northern climate, we have developed a sun-worshipping culture. The sun is warm, comforting and inviting, and we eagerly await the summer months, when life seems easier and we can spend time outdoors. But the message that health authorities around the world are trying to get across should not be ignored. In plain terms, all the research points to one thing: sunlight may make you feel good, but the sun can kill.

Does that sound a bit dramatic? It's no exaggeration. Last year over 40,000 people in the UK got skin cancer; 32,000 of these cases could have been prevented if the sufferers had behaved differently in the sun. The number of skin-cancer victims is doubling every ten years, and this huge rise coincides with the twentieth century fashion for a tan. Our protection from the sun is decreasing at an alarming rate, partly because of the thinning of the ozone layer. Our summers are also getting hotter, thanks to global warming. We have to consider the fact that we aren't really a typical 'northern' clime any longer, and it's time to take lessons from our neighbours further south. In hotter climates, locals practise behaviour they have learnt in order to survive: they get up earlier, take a siesta after lunch, and wear cotton clothes in dark colours that absorb ultraviolet rays. And in most cases, these people have the advantage of darker skin, which is more protective against the harmful effects of the sun.

Sheree Murphy
✿ Before going to bed I always put a bit of spot cream on my face in those little problem areas around my chin. This seems to prevent spots from coming.
✿ As I have long hair I always use conditioner and once a month I use a 20-minute leave-in conditioner, just to give it that extra boost.
✿ I use a product called serum very sparingly in my hair before blow-drying it. This stops it from being frizzy and flyaway.
✿ When I lived at home my mum used to trim my hair every two weeks. This kept it really healthy and I never had a split end. I would recommend regular cutting if you have long hair, as it really can get straggly and damaged if left too long.

WHAT'S THE REAL RISK?

Skin cancer is caused by ultraviolet radiation from the sun, or sunbeds. Ultraviolet radiation is divided into three bands, UVA, UVB and UVC, depending on how much energy they have. UVC, with the most energy, is the most harmful, but the ozone layer screens it out. UVB does the most damage to your skin and causes skin cancer. UVA penetrates deeper into the skin than UVB and causes premature ageing. In fact, the sun causes a full 90 per cent of the ageing we see on our skin, in the form of wrinkles, dark spots, sagging skin (sunlight reduces the skin's elasticity) and red, rough patches. Experts say that there is no such thing as a healthy tan – once those rays hit your body, the damage is done.

There are three types of skin cancer. The two most common are 'basal cell' and 'squamous cell' carcinoma. Poor tanners, especially those with red hair and freckles, are most at risk of basal cell carcinoma. Outdoor workers and the over-fifties, who have built up a lifetime's exposure to the sun, are most at risk of squamous cell carcinoma. These cancers are largely curable, but they can be seriously disfiguring.

The third type of skin cancer is the most dangerous and, frighteningly, is far more likely to affect young people. Melanoma is the third most common cancer among women aged 15 to 34. Melanoma is normally first noticed when a mole or freckle grows, or changes shape or colour, growing aggressively downwards. If it is caught in time, it can be cut out, but advanced melanoma spreads quickly to the liver, bones, lungs and brain. Once it has spread, there is no cure.

PRACTISE SAFE SUN

Avoid the fiercest heat of the day, wearing a hat and loose, tightly-woven, dark cotton clothing that covers your arms and legs as well as your body. You can still get sunburnt under a beach umbrella, under water, in the shade and on hazy days (up to 80 per cent of the sun's rays reach earth even when the sky is overcast), so wear a high SPF sunscreen and other protective gear even when the weather is gloomy.

The beneficial effects of sunshine are as powerful early in the morning and the evening as they are in the heat of the day, and you'll run less risk of suffering other debilitating effects of the hot weather: sunstroke, sunburn and prickly heat.

Even dark skins wrinkle badly after prolonged exposure to the sun. In skins unused to the sun, exposure produces heat redness, and even blistering. Gradual exposure, with a good SPF suncream, encourages the skin to step up melanin production, which gives natural protection against sunburn. In fair skins which have little melanin-producing capacity, exposure can produce malignant changes – in other words, cancer. Most of us have had a sunburn – in fact, in the 80s it was believed that the best way to tan was to burn repeatedly to encourage a darker tan. We now know that just two cases of severe sunburn in childhood can double your risk of skin cancer in later life. Avoid sunburn at all costs.

If you are caught out, and sunburn is the result, there are things you can do to limit the damage:

- Take the homeopathic remedy sol (30c) every four hours, for up to ten doses to relieve the effects.
- Aloe vera gel or urtica urens ointment (available from a good health shop) will ease the pain and help to prevent skin damage.
- Rescue remedy cream, a Bach flower remedy, works to heal damaged tissue and reduce discomfort.
- Take a cool bath to help take the heat out of the burn. Wear loose clothing and drink plenty of fresh water. Avoid the sun entirely until all traces of burning have disappeared.

BENEFITS WITHOUT RISKS

Despite the bad press, suntans are still in style. Until we, as a culture, get smart and bring back the vogue for an 'English rose' complexion, the best way to attain the in look is to fake it. There is a wide variety of 'self-tanning' creams, sprays and lotions on the market – many of which contain extra nutrients for the skin as well as sunscreens. For suntan devotees, this is the safest way to go bronze.

HEALTHY HAIR

Once again, it's inside out. If you have a good diet, with lots of fresh foods containing the essential vitamins, minerals and other nutrients, your hair will reflect your health. Over-blow-drying, sun damage and chemical processing (perms and colouring, for example) can cause problems, including dry hair, split ends, frizziness and discoloration, but you can remedy much of these by applying conditioners regularly and keeping your hair clean.

HAIRCARE TIPS

- Sun, heat, chlorine, hair colouring, over-drying and product build-up all play havoc with the health and appearance of our hair.
- Hard water, with a high mineral content, can be hard on hair. It neither lathers up nor rinses out easily, so it may leave your hair feeling less than sparkling-clean. Hard water may react chemically with coloured or processed hair, especially blonde or red. It can turn it brassy or aqua-ish. Consider a charcoal-based shower filter that takes out the minerals that cause the most damage. In the US there are now shampoo concentrates for different water types – they are bound to hit our markets soon.
- Never brush wet hair or tug at tangles.
- Brushing dry hair will stimulate clogged scalps and lift out grime.
- Set your blow-dryer on low and quit before that bone-dry stage. Blast with cool air to seal in the moisture.
- Don't pull your hair too tight with bands, pins or clips, and avoid sharp-edges.
- If your hair is coloured or processed, the above tips are even more important.
- As we get older, our hair and scalp may get drier. To keep them looking healthy, use a conditioner each time you shampoo, and let your hair air-dry once in a while, instead of using a blow-dryer.

SOME REMEDIES TO MAKE AT HOME

Anti-cellulite Scrub

30 ml/2 tbsp finely ground lentils
15 ml/1 tbsp coarse ground oatmeal
15 ml/1 tbsp grapeseed oil
30 ml/2 tbsp witch hazel
6 drops juniper oil

This treatment will encourage your circulation to shift stubborn cellulite. Blend the ingredients to form a thick paste. Using the palms of your hands, firmly massage the mixture across the thighs, hips and buttocks. Rub the surface of the skin in circular motions, massaging the entire area for at least three minutes. Shower off with alternate blasts of cool and icy water.

Moisture Mask

½ ripe avocado
5 ml/1 tsp honey
1 egg yolk

This is an ideal mask for dry or mature skin. Mix all the ingredients together and apply to a clean throat and face. Relax for 15 minutes while the skin absorbs the nourishing ingredients. Avocados have the highest oil and protein content of any fruit and are rich in antioxidant vitamins (see page 26). Egg yolk is the richest source of lecithin, which can lock moisture into the skin.

Anti-ageing facial oil

25m1/1 oz almond oil
25 ml/1 oz jojoba oil
5 evening primrose oil capsules (contents)
10 drops wheatgerm oil
10 drops frankincense oil (or geranium)

Use this rich oil at night to fortify and rejuvenate your skin. It's a great alternative to expensive skin scrubs.

Oily- and combination-skin scrub

7.5 ml/½ tbsp ground almonds
25 ml/1½ tbsp medium ground oatmeal
5ml/1 tsp fresh lemon juice
water to mix

This solution will help to deep-clean the skin and discourage spots and blackheads. Use it three times a week, but be careful not to rub too hard, or it will over-excite your sebaceous glands.

ANTI-AGEING TECHNIQUES

Scientists are now able to pinpoint the physical indications of ageing, and the various stages at which they occur, and to some extent are able to ascertain why they occur. While experts still do not understand why we age, and why degeneration in the body occurs, they do know what causes some of the problems normally associated with ageing, and are able to retard or halt the degenerative processes associated with them.

We age in a variety of ways, some of which are very visible, including a decline in height, shrinkage of muscle, thinning and greying of hair, and wrinkling of skin.

Although there is no doubt that we will all age – for there is nothing to stop the passage of time – there are ways to lessen the effect.

SELF-HELP

■ If you use a sunscreen daily, your body will repair some of the damage caused by earlier exposure, and you'll look younger. Sunscreen prevents age spots, wrinkles and skin cancer.

Energizing bath oil
5 drops peppermint oil
3 drops neroli oil
2 drops jasmine oil

Add to the bath and wait to be picked up!

After-sun soothing oil
50ml/2 fl oz grapeseed oil
50m1/2 fl oz virgin olive oil
15ml/1 tbsp wheatgerm oil
10 drops chamomile essential oil

You can repair some of the damage caused by the sun's rays with this nourishing oil. It has a high vitamin E content, and will help to reverse the ageing effects of overexposure to the sun.

Oil for problem nails
50ml/2 fl oz almond oil
15 drops tea tree oil
10 drops bergamot oil

Massage this oil into your nails twice daily if you suffer from dry or discoloured nails, inflammation or fungal infections.

Dry-ends sealer
25m1/1½ tbsp almond oil
25ml/1½ tbsp olive oil
25m1/1½ tbsp apricot or peach kernel oil
5 drops wheatgerm oil

Mix the oils together and apply a tiny quantity to the ends of your hair. It will temporarily seal split ends and nourish the hair above them.

Dry hair conditioner
½ ripe avocado
1 egg yolk
5ml/1 tsp fresh lemon juice
60ml/4 tbsp olive oil

Beat the egg in a food processor or in a blender. Slowly add the oil until it reaches the consistency of mayonnaise. Stir in the finely mashed pulp of the avocado and the lemon juice. Coat the hair in the 'mayonnaise', and work it into the scalp. Wrap the head in a hot towel to keep in body heat and promote greater absorption. Leave for at least half an hour before rinsing with just-warm water. Use a milk shampoo to remove all remaining traces. Use once a month.

- Most leafy green and brightly coloured vegetables contain a substance called beta carotene, a type of Vitamin A which acts as an antioxidant (see page 26) and has been proved to help prevent, and in some cases reverse, the effects of ageing.
- Fruit and vegetables rich in vitamin C improve overall health, and the antioxidant benefits can help to retard the ageing process. Eat plenty of citrus fruits, red peppers, cabbage, tomatoes, spinach and broccoli.
- Drink plenty of water. Water hydrates your system, ensures the speedy elimination of toxins, acts as a mild diuretic and cleanses the body.
- A high-fibre diet stimulates the digestive tract, and makes elimination more efficient. You are much less likely to get spots and skin problems if your bowels are working properly.
- One of the greatest causes of ageing is stress, which places incredible physical, mental and psychological demands on our bodies. Stress

has now been linked to premature ageing, high blood pressure, heart disease, and niggling ailments that we associate with age, including skin complaints. See page 45 for ways to cope with stress.

- Evidence proves that both the mind and body benefit from a good night's sleep, which ensures you perform at optimum levels and improve your appearance. The greatest concentration of growth hormones are released at night, and these help the body to repair and rejuvenate.
- Avoid smoking, which causes wrinkles, reduces lung capacity (making it more difficult to get oxygen to those needy cells) and is a primary cause of cancer.
- Be happy. The strong relationship between the mind and the body means that when you feel great, you'll look great and you'll be more likely to achieve optimum health.

SKIN PROBLEMS

The causes of skin problems can be very difficult to identify. They are often a complex combination of diet, environment, general health, hereditary factors, stress and individual susceptibility. The length of time it takes to cure a skin complaint will largely depend on how long medicated ointments or drugs have been used to suppress the condition in the past, and the state of your other organs. Almost all the modern-day 'cures' for skin problems aren't, in fact, cures at all. They work by easing symptoms so that we look and feel better, but rarely do anything about the cause of the condition. Stop taking your medication, and the problem crops up again. To successfully cure a skin problem, you have to go a step further – find out what's causing it and then address that cause, whether it's linked to your diet, your lifestyle, an allergy or a genetic tendency towards that kind of

Malandra Burrows
✿ Always moisturize well to keep your skin healthy and supple.
✿ Your skin reflects your overall health, so a good diet, exercise and plenty of water will keep your skin healthy.
✿ I take cod liver oil every day and I find that this really helps my skin's vitality.
✿ Choose a moisturizer with UV protection for use all year round. The sun has a very drying and ageing effect on the skin.
✿ Try to choose products that are unperfumed and simple, as these will be less harsh on your skin.

problem.

The remedies suggested here will improve most skin conditions, but for deep-seated skin problems, finding a real cure can take time, and may only be possible by working at it with the help of a professional therapist: homeopaths, nutritional therapists and Chinese herbalists are a good bet for skin problems.

WHAT GOES WRONG

In natural medicine, skin conditions, which include those affecting hair and nails, are viewed as manifestations of general imbalance and poor functioning of the body processes. Skin tone and colour tell a therapist a great deal about a person.

ACNE

Acne is characterized by blackheads and pustules, normally found on the face and back. This problem is linked with hormonally-induced hyperactivity of the oil-producing glands.

WHAT CAN YOU DO?

- There is a dietary factor in acne related to how well the body can metabolize fats and carbohydrates. Although greasy foods don't actually cause acne, it's a good idea to cut down on fats, sweets and refined carbohydrates, which your body may have trouble processing. Eat more fresh fruit and vegetables, and drink as much pure water as you can manage.
- Skin cleansing is an important aspect of the treatment of acne, and regular facial steams are a good way of healing the skin and cleansing the pores without adding more grease. Use a few drops of the following essential oils in hot water for a facial steam: bergamot, chamomile, lavender or lemon grass. These oils may also be well diluted in

olive oil and massaged into the skin.

- Try some herbs to cleanse the body: burdock root, cleavers, echinacca and yellow dock are good, and can be taken in tablet form, or drunk as a decoction (boiled in water). Take three times a day for several weeks.
- Once the acne has cleared up, massage comfrey ointment into the old sites of the spots to help reduce scarring.

ECZEMA

The symptoms of eczema include redness, flakiness and weeping skin. It may start as tiny blisters that burst and leave a red, raw surface. The incidence of eczema has increased dramatically in recent years, especially among children. People with eczema often suffer also from hayfever and asthma.

WHAT CAN YOU DO?

Curing eczema using natural remedies is possible, but it takes time. If a cure requires general 'detoxification', the eczema may get worse before it gets better, as the body struggles to eliminate more through the skin, and generally becomes healthier.

- A combination of herbs, drunk as an infusion (added to boiling water and steeped like tea), will help to relieve inflammation and cleanse the body. Try burdock, chamomile, heartsease, marigold or red clover, three times a day for six weeks. Take a two-week break and start again.
- Use chickweed or calendula ointments on affected areas.
- Watch out for foods that exacerbate the condition. It may be caused by an intolerance or allergy to wheat or dairy produce, for example, or even citrus fruits or any other foods. If you notice your condition becomes worse after eating some things, cut them out for a week to see if there is an improvement.
- If your eczema is caused by or related to stress, try a relaxation therapy, and get some regular exercise to help reduce stress levels. A daily aromatherapy bath with lavender oil or melissa may help.
- Take extra vitamins B, C and zinc, and add

safflower or evening primrose oil capsules to your diet.

- Try the homeopathic remedy graphites for eczema that mainly affects the palms of the hands and the area behind the ears. Skin that is red, dry, rough and itchy, aggravated by heat and washing, may respond to sulphur. For skin that cracks easily, the homeopathic remedy petroleum may help. Take them four times daily for two weeks. If you don't see any results, consult a professional homeopath.

Freya Copeland

✿ As soon as you can after work I recommend taking off your make-up, as it clogs the pores and dries out the skin.

✿ I always carry a lip balm in nearly every pocket I have. I am obsessed with the stuff; I hate having dry lips. Carry one around with you and get yourself luscious lips!

✿ Make sure you cover yourself from top to toe with lovely moisturizing lotion every day. This will make your whole body feel smooth and soft.

✿ If you have long hair and you are bored to death with it get it chopped off! I don't regret having mine cut. I feel much more like 'Freya' now and it takes only seconds to do in the morning.

✿ When you go for a big night out make sure you wear lashings of mascara and to make your eyes appear even wider, apply a little soft eye pencil at the corners.

PSORIASIS

Psoriasis is a common skin disease in which red, scaly spots and patches appear on the skin of the bony areas of the body, such as elbows, eyebrows or scalp. The patches occur because the body is over-producing skin cells in those areas. The skin tends to flake off from the affected area, which can become itchy.

The condition can be triggered by shock or trauma, and flare-ups often occur during stressful times of life. The symptoms are often alleviated by sunshine and swimming in the sea.

WHAT CAN YOU DO?

Psoriasis is notoriously difficult to treat by any kind of medicine. Severe cases will often be considerably improved by natural remedies, and children tend to be easier to cure.

- Herbs that help to clear psoriasis out of the system include burdock, sarsaparilla and yellow dock root, which can be drunk three times daily for up to three months.
- An ointment made of comfrey root can be massaged into the patches to help reduce flaking.
- Essential oils can be diluted in olive oil and massaged into the patches to improve skin and reduce scaling. Try bergamot, lavender and sandalwood.
- Providing you do not have sensitive skin, careful sunbathing (six sessions, at ten minutes each) may help to clear up an outbreak.
- Take extra zinc in your diet, and betacarotene.
- The homeopathic remedy sulphur will help if your skin is dry, red, scaly, with itchy patches that are worse after baths. Arsenicum is useful if the affected areas of the skin are burning hot, and you feel chilly. Petroleum is good when the condition is aggravated by cold and worse in the winter.

OVERALL

Recent research shows that antioxidants, called the age-erasing nutrients, can prevent the degenerative processes of ageing. Most researchers have focused their attention on the effects of vitamins C, E and betacarotene, as well as the mineral selenium. Studies show that high dosages of these nutrients result in low incidences of disease and, particularly relevant here, slow the ageing process of skin and other body organs. Experts recommend that you get

> ➤ **UNDERSTANDING SUN PROTECTION FACTORS (SPFS)**
>
> Everyone should wear sunscreens with a high SPF. As a rule of thumb, multiply the SPF number by the length of time you can normally stay in the sun without burning to find out how long you are safe to be in full sunlight. For example, a fair-skinned blonde may bum in 20 minutes of full sunlight. If you want to spend an afternoon in the sun (say 5 hours), you will need SPF 15 (20 minutes x 15 = 300 minutes, or five hours), and probably SPF20 to 30 in the hottest months. Darker-skinned people should use SPF6–8 daily, and SPF15 outdoors in the summer.

all or as many of your RDAs (recommended daily allowances) as possible of each antioxidant from the food you eat. For added protection, take between 100 and 400IU (international units) of vitamin E, between 500 and 1,000 mg of vitamin C and between six and 30 mg beta-carotene. Selenium can be taken at 30 mg. Zinc and copper will also help skin conditions, and can be taken as part of a good multi-vitamin supplement. There are many supplements available specially for hair and nails, and they can be taken alongside your normal vitamin and mineral supplement.

Take care of your skin on a daily basis, think about what you put into your body and how it will affect its functioning. Don't forget that the skin is a mirror of your health. If it's showing signs of stress, an unhealthy lifestyle or an inadequate diet, now is the time to do something about it. Healthy skin looks beautiful and, most importantly, gives you confidence. To paraphrase an old saying, put your best face forward.

DANDRUFF

Dandruff occurs when the fine cells of the outer layer of skin on the scalp are shed at a faster rate than normal, causing the characteristic flakes of dead skin. This is caused by a disorder of the sebaceous glands. If too little sebum is secreted, the hair is dry and dandruff appears as white flakes; if too much sebum is produced, the hair is greasy, and the dandruff yellow. The flakes are usually most obvious after brushing or combing the hair, which loosens them.

One of the following homeopathic remedies might help. Take one 6x tablet two or three times daily for two weeks. If you don't see any improvement, see a homeopath for specialist advice.

- Arsenicum for dry, sensitive, hot scalp with bare patches.
- Natrum mur for white crust around hairline and greasy hair.
- Fluonic acid for flaky scalp and hair loss.
- Graphites for a moist scalp with smelly crusting.
- Sulphur for thick dandruff that is itchier at night.
- Sepia for moist, greasy scalp, sensitive around the ears.
- Dilute lavender essential oil in a little almond or coconut oil and massage into the scalp to eliminate dandruff.

Increase your intake of:
- Selenium
- Vitamin E
- Vitamin C
- B-complex vitamins
- Zinc
- Rosemary is an excellent herb for dandruff because it improves the circulation to the scalp. You can take it internally, or use it as an application. For dry hair, add a couple of drops of rosemary essential oil to some olive oil and rub it into the scalp before washing. For greasy hair, add rosemary vinegar or a few drops of rosemary essential oil to the rinsing water.

BALDING
About 85 per cent of balding is hereditary. Men first lose their hair on the crown and at the hairline, while women are more likely to lose hair evenly over the entire scalp. No one is quite sure what causes hair to stop growing, but it may be caused by the male hormone testosterone. When balding is hereditary, there isn't a great deal you can do about it. There are some remedies (suggested below) that might help, but once it starts hair loss is difficult to stop. There are, however, many non-hereditary factors that can cause hair to thin, including long-term stress, or a traumatic event such as divorce or bereavement, fad diets that don't give you enough protein, anaemia, childbirth, drugs (including birth control, steroids, beta blockers and those derived from vitamin A), lupus, arthritis and a poor diet.

Here are some remedies for both types of balding:

The following homeopathic remedies can help in specific cases. Take two 6c tablets daily for three to four weeks. If you do not see any change in either the rate of loss or regrowth, contact a registered practitioner for specialist advice.
- Lycopodium for hair loss after childbirth.
- Aurum for hair loss with headaches and boils on the scalp.
- Phosphonic acid for hair loss after grief, and with exhaustion.
- Arnica for hair loss after injury.
- Selenium for painful scalp and loss of body hair along with hair on head.
- Sepia for hair loss related to menopause or childbirth.

Increase your intake of:
- Vitamin B-complex (high-dosage tablet, twice daily)
- Choline
- Inositol
- Calcium
- Magnesium
- Vitamins and minerals in a good supplement.

Chinese Herbalism is widely used to treat hair loss, including that associated with pattern or hereditary balding. You'll need to see a registered practitioner for treatment, but the following patent remedies are believed to be effective in many cases.
- Shou Wu Pian is commonly used in China to keep hair from greying, and to prevent hair loss.
- In Chinese medicine, hair loss is attributed to deficient liver and kidneys and specific herbs to address this include wolfberry, mulberry and fleece flower root. Your herbalist can prepare a treatment that will work for you.

An old folk remedy for baldness is sage tea. Drink it twice a day – who knows, it might work!

6. The Natural Way to Health

WE ARE IN the middle of a healthcare revolution. After decades of placing our health in the hands of conventional medicine, we are ringing in the changes. We have begun to listen to our bodies, and to take some responsibility for our own health. Conventional medicine is great – it's there for serious illnesses and it can perform miracles for many of our modern-day health problems. However, there are drawbacks, and that is why we have begun to explore some of the options in the complementary field. For example, conventional medicine has only just begun to pay attention to holistic health – that is, treating the mind, body and spirit together, rather than treating just the physical symptoms of ill-health. We have talked earlier about the powerful mind – body relationship, and complementary medicine takes that very seriously, basing treatment on the whole you, rather than just the parts that aren't working properly.

There are many conditions for which conventional medicine has no cure – for example, eczema, asthma, irritable bowel syndrome, allergies and much, much more. Sure, it offers drugs, but these do little other than suppress the symptoms to make us feel better. The condition still exists, underneath the relief of symptoms. That's where complementary medicine is also different. Complementary treatments address the root cause of a problem, for example, an overstretched immune system in the case of allergies, or stress in the case of chronic, unexplained headaches.

Eight out of ten people in the UK have now used a complementary treatment in some form, and the numbers are increasing. Apart from the fact that they can be much more effective for some conditions than conventional medicine, complementary treatments allow us to take some control, which can also encourage the healing process. There is something very satisfying about considering our own health needs and then taking steps to treat ourselves, with a little professional help, using the ever-increasing range of natural medicines.

After all the health scares of the past few years, including the overuse of antibiotics and the growing concern about the level of side-effects caused by drugs, many of us are exploring natural alternatives that work with the body to encourage it to heal itself.

There are literally hundreds of different remedies and treatments now available. Some of them you can practise at home with a little knowledge. Others you'll need to see a practitioner to use correctly and effectively. Most of the remedies are inexpensive – less expensive, for example, than a prescription, and some of the therapies, such as acupuncture, homeopathy and osteopathy, can sometimes be paid for by a private health insurance scheme, and increasingly often by the NHS. Most therapies are not expensive if you take into consideration the fact that treatment will, in many cases, reduce your need for drugs and probably alleviate the condition completely. It's a great investment of both your time and money.

Alternative therapies should not be considered a replacement for conventional medicine, but should work hand in hand with it to prevent illness and ensure that your body is working at optimum level so that when you do get ill, you heal quickly, and without intervention. Save the doctor for those illnesses that can't be treated outside the surgery, where modern medicine can make all the difference.

Alternative therapies are vastly different, and may call upon the medical practices of other cultures which treat illness and health in a completely different way.

WHICH THERAPY IS RIGHT FOR YOU?

The variety of therapies available makes it very difficult to choose which one is best for you. Many of the therapies, such as ayurveda, homeopathy, acupuncture and reflexology, are systems of medicine which include diet, lifestyle and medical attention and, for a beginner, or someone with a chronic, long-standing health problem, these might prove to be the most useful, outlining exactly how to change habits in order to achieve optimum health and well-being.

If you cringe at the thought of needles, acupuncture may not be for you, but acupressure, which involves working the same points with pressure rather than needles, may be more suitable. If you are hopeless at remembering to take tablets, something like aromatherapy might be more useful than, say, homeopathy or Chinese herbalism.

Many therapies can be combined, for example, aromatherapy is complementary to most other therapies except homeopathy, which may be affected by some of the more powerful oils.

Alyson Spiro
✿ *I use a lot of different homeopathic remedies with the children. One of my favourites, due to its effectiveness, is arnica, which brings down bruising and swelling.*
✿ *Chinese herbs are a great favourite of mine and although a lot of them are really nasty to drink, I really do believe they aided my husband's and my fertility. I also took them all the way through pregnancy and they made me feel very well indeed.*

All the Chinese treatments (acupuncture, herbalism, Chi Gung and acupressure, among others) work well together. As a rule of thumb, try one therapy at a time so you know which one works for you. Add others when you've found one that keeps you happy. You may find that Chinese herbalism controls your eczema, but you like to have your spirits lifted by the occasional osteopathic treatment, or aromatherapy bath. That's perfectly acceptable. The whole point of alternative therapies is that you are taking charge of your own health, and by ensuring that your sense of well-being is the best it can be, you will be on course to attain good health on every level.

WHAT TO EXPECT FROM ALTERNATIVE THERAPIES

Alternative therapies approach things in a completely different way to conventional medicine. You will be expected to give details of everything about you and your health in order for your therapist to make an informed decision about treatment. Your symptoms will not be treated, rather their root cause will be investigated and dealt with. You can expect, occasionally, for your symptoms to become worse before they get better, which is a sign that your body is responding to treatment and beginning to help itself. The basis of all alternative therapies is that they stimulate your body to heal itself.

WARNING

Medical emergencies must always be addressed by a qualified doctor. Alternative medicine is not a replacement for conventional medicine, but a complement to it. Make sure you tell your GP about any alternative treatments you are receiving, and tell your alternative health practitioner about any conventional medication.

DO ALTERNATIVE THERAPIES WORK?

There is a great deal of contemporary research into the efficacy of alternative therapies. There is no question that most of them do work, although modern science has had difficulty in justifying that on a scientific level. Healing, for instance, works for thousands and thousands of people each year, and in some cases terminal illnesses have been cured. There is no explanation for how this has happened but we do know that it has. Some people believe that alternative therapies

work because there is so much time spent in consultation with the practitioner, which is, in itself, therapeutic. But this doesn't explain the fact that most of the therapies listed in this book work on infants, babies and people who are no longer able to think for themselves. Some therapies will work for you, some may not. Experiment and enjoy the process.

SAFETY NOTES

Some therapies are not suitable for certain age groups and health conditions. Some aromatherapy oils can bring on contractions, which could cause miscarriage in a pregnant woman. Certain bone diseases must never be treated with osteopathy or chiropractic. Your practitioner must be aware of any and all health conditions you suffer from in order to advise the best possible treatment.

Babies, children and the elderly will all respond to the majority of therapies, depending on the severity of their condition, although some are more suitable than others. Conditions like colic and hyperactivity in children, menopausal complaints, degenerative diseases, and many others, have no conventional cures, but they have been successfully treated with alternative therapies.

CHOOSING A PRACTITIONER

The success of alternative therapies can be enormously dependent on a good practitioner – patient relationship, and your choice of a therapist is as important as the choice of therapy. Take your time, check the therapist's qualifications and do not commit yourself until you are sure you can build a rapport. Because you will be imparting a great deal of information about yourself to the therapist, who must be able to take it on board and diagnose and treat you on that basis, you must feel comfortable with your chosen practitioner, and feel able to be honest about yourself and your complaint.

The following steps will help you in your choice:

■ Ask your GP or other therapist for a recommendation.
■ Ring the organization or association of the therapy you are interested in for a list of practitioners.

- Speak to your practitioner on the telephone in the first instance.
- If you are happy with what they say, make an appointment.
- Ask to see his or her qualifications before committing yourself.
- Establish whether or not you feel you will be able to get along with the therapist, in particular whether you think you will be able to 'relate'. Instinct is of prime importance here.
- Be sure that you have confidence in the practitioner, and that he or she is supportive and helpful but not intrusive.
- Find out if your therapist has any experience in treating the condition from which you suffer, and how he or she went about it.
- If you are happy with all these things, go ahead with the consultation.

Remember that prices vary enormously between therapists, and some therapies can be expensive. Be sure you know what you are getting for your money before committing yourself to anything.

THE CONSULTATION

The consultation is the most important part of any alternative therapy session. This is the first session with a therapist, and the one in which the most information is exchanged. The first session usually lasts longer than any subsequent sessions because your therapist will aim to find out all about you as well as your problem before any diagnosis can be made. You can expect your therapist to ask you all about:

- Your physical condition, including past and present illnesses, any medication you are taking, any symptoms and interesting aspects to them (are there sharp pains, or do they come on in the morning).
- Your diet, including cravings, appetite, any weight problems, alcohol intake.
- Your sleep patterns.
- Job and home life, whether or not you have children, a partner, or any obvious stresses.
- Your exercise patterns.
- Your emotional state – are things making you unhappy? Have you recently moved, split up with a partner, lost someone

significant, failed an important exam?
- Any other treatment you may be undergoing, either conventional and complementary.
- What you hope to get from treatment.

With this information, your therapist can go ahead and make a diagnosis.

DIAGNOSTIC TECHNIQUES

Each discipline has different techniques for finalizing the diagnosis. In Chinese medicine, for instance, your practitioner will look at your tongue, take a number of pulses, palpate your body, and assess you by looking at different parts of your body. With that information, and the facts gleaned from the original information-gathering session, he will prescribe a course of treatment.

Some therapies use X-rays to aid diagnosis, others use iridology (looking at the eyes as a map of the body and pinpointing any weaknesses in the irises), others use diagnostic techniques such as:
- Kinesiology (muscle tests which display the health of the whole body).
- Kirlian photography (photographing the quality of the energy of a person or object, which is altered where there is imbalance or illness).
- Biofeedback (monitoring responses to various physical tests by machine).

Many physical therapies will be able to locate problem areas in the process of an examination. A reflexologist will, for instance, be able to tell a lot about your physical condition by your response to her finger pressure on your feet. Sensitivity indicates an imbalance in the related systems. Other, less physical systems, such as homeopathy, may all be done on the basis of your verbal communication, which makes it all the more important for you to be honest with your therapist.

HOW TO JUDGE THE RESULTS

Many people do not seek out alternative therapies until they have become thoroughly disillusioned by conventional medicine, and by then many long-standing conditions have become quite deeply entrenched. It is normal for treatments to take some time. These are not miracle cures, but gentle and effective means of encouraging your body to work for itself. For example, it is normally believed that it takes as long to treat eczema as the length of time you have suffered from the condition.

Many therapies initiate a process of detoxification, which means that toxins are forced out of the body. When this happens, you may suffer from symptoms such as headaches, dizziness, bad skin, rashes, diarrhoea, nausea and discharge. This is normal, and symptoms should never be so uncomfortable as to be unbearable. You may find that symptoms become worse or change as your treatment progresses. This is also normal, and it shows that your body is hard at work.

If you experience no change in your condition, or you are feeling much worse, chances are the treatment is not working and you should go back to your therapist. Always give your therapist a second chance; diagnosis is extremely complicated and you may, unknowingly, have omitted a major piece of information that changes the whole treatment. If several attempts to effect a cure fail completely, you may think about trying a different therapy, or a different therapist. Remember that it will take time, and your therapist can only be as good as the information you have given him or her.

COMPLAINTS PROCEDURES

All therapies have governing bodies and associations which usually try to ensure the reputation of their discipline. They will have names of registered, qualified therapists, and if you have a complaint, the regulatory board will deal with it. Some therapies do not require professional qualifications, but all good therapists should be able to show evidence of their training, and belong to a recognized board. If your therapist does not belong to one, write a letter to their training college or faculty. If you are genuinely unhappy with treatment, your money should be refunded.

A GUIDE TO THERAPIES

The following is a very basic introduction to some of the most popular therapies. It's beyond the scope of this book to go into any more detail, but it will help you to decide whether or not a therapy is for you. If you are keen to try one of the therapies listed, contact their regulatory board (see useful addresses), who will help you to find a practitioner in your area.

Alyson Spiro

✿ *My sister is a hypnotherapist and she helped me with some visualization techniques which helped me get through the pain of labour.*

✿ *One of my children was a forceps delivery, and I took her for cranial osteopathy. She was quite traumatized and I would recommend it because a lot of the tension around her skull was released and she became much better.*

ACUPUNCTURE

Acupuncture is based on the idea that we have a vital life force, 'chi', that runs through meridians in our bodies. Using fine needles, your therapist will gently work at key points along these meridians to balance, improve the flow of energy, and address organs and systems that are affected by each meridian. Meridians run through many parts of the body, and every point along a specific meridian will be affected by disharmony at any other point. For example, the teeth are part of the stomach meridian, and teething problems may affect the length of the meridian, including the stomach; and as a result many babies suffer digestive disorders as part of the condition.

Sometimes your acupuncturist might use 'moxa', a herb that can be burnt at acupuncture points across the body. There are various other tools and techniques used.

Treats: stress, depression, pain relief, addictions, childbirth, ME, allergies, asthma and eczema, injuries, fatigue, digestive disorders, circulatory disorders, menstrual problems, sexual problems, infertility.

Acupressure involves the use of finger pressure on acupuncture points to stimulate the smooth flow of chi through the energy channels of the body. It involves mostly thumb and fingertip pressure, although it can also incorporate massage along the meridians.

ALEXANDER TECHNIQUE
The Alexander Technique, created by Frederick Alexander, an Australian actor, focuses on the fundamental belief that by correcting the way the body is held and used, physical and psychological well-being can be enhanced. The Alexander Technique is not a therapy as such, but a process of re-education, which allows us to rediscover our natural poise, grace and freedom, and use our bodies more efficiently. It is often referred to as 'posture training', and it is taught in lessons where the practitioner is referred to as a teacher. Overall, the Alexander Technique is aimed at encouraging awareness of your body, so that you have an increased sense of confidence, greater vitality, and an improved, positive mental outlook. Improved physical health will also result.

Treats: sessions are aimed at improving overall posture and body, responses, and many conditions respond to this, particularly asthma, headaches, eczema and fatigue, all of which are exacerbated by stress. Overall, circulatory problems, breathing disorders, musculo-skeletal conditions may respond to treatment, although it does not set out to 'cure' as such, rather to encourage the body's systems to work more effectively.

AROMATHERAPY
Aromatherapy uses essential oils – the 'life force' of aromatic flowers, herbs, plants, trees or spices – for therapeutic purposes. Each oil has its own individual qualities which affect physical and psychological well-being. The therapeutic properties of the essential oils are able to work towards restoring a harmonious balance within the body so that it is able to function more effectively. There are special forms of massage specifically designed for use with aromatherapy, and when these oils come into contact with the skin, they stimulate nerve endings, circulation, the lymphatic system, muscles, tissues, the nervous system, and endocrine activity, according to their specific qualities. When oils are inhaled, they stimulate nerve endings in the nose and messages are carried to the brain in this way. Occasionally oils are prescribed for internal use. Aromatherapy oils can be used in massage, the bath, steam inhalations, vaporizers, compresses, creams, gargles, mouthwashes, douches and sometimes taken neat.

Treats: aromatherapy is a holistic therapy. For this reason, almost any health condition can be improved by general use. It is extremely effective for stress and related disorders, muscular problems, emotional disorders, female complaints such as menopause, pregnancy and period problems, digestive disorders and skin problems.

AYURVEDIC MEDICINE
Ayurvedic medicine is the traditional, all-embracing national system of medicine practised in India and Sri Lanka. Like traditional Chinese medicine, Ayurveda is a comprehensive system of healthcare with many elements working together to provide guidance for living; it is a way of life, rather than a treatment for specific illnesses. Some of the elements of Ayurvedic medicine include:
- a type of aromatherapy
- breathing
- detoxification
- diet
- exercise
- herbs
- manipulation of vital energy points (called marma)
- meditation
- music therapy
- techniques aimed at emotional and psychological health
- yoga

The basic Ayurvedic belief is that everything within the universe, including ourselves, is composed of energy or 'prana'. By balancing that energy within ourselves and in relation to the world around us, we will promote health on

TOP TEN AROMATHERAPY OILS

The following oils are great for the majority of health conditions, and are ideal to have at home for day-to-day use.

Clary Sage
Properties: warming, soothing, aphrodisiac.
Uses: menstrual problems, depression, anxiety, high blood pressure.

Eucalyptus
Properties: antiseptic, decongestant, antiviral.
Uses: colds, chest infections, aches and pains.

Geranium
Properties: soothing, refreshing, relaxing, antidepressant, astringent.
Uses: PMS, menopause, apathy, anxiety, skin complaints.

Lavender
Properties: soothing, antiseptic, generally therapeutic.
Uses: skin problems, insomnia, stress, indigestion, cystitis, headache, burns.

Lemon
Properties: refreshing, antiseptic, stimulating.
Uses: warts, depression, acne, indigestion.

Peppermint
Properties: digestive, cooling, refreshing, mentally stimulating.
Uses: muscle fatigue, bad breath, toothache, bronchitis, indigestion, travel sickness.

Petitgrain
Properties: soothing, calming, antidepressant.
Uses: skin problems, apathy, irritability, depression.

Rosemary
Properties: stimulating, refreshing.
Uses: muscle fatigue, colds, poor circulation, aches and pains, mental fatigue.

Tea tree
Properties: anti-fungal, antiseptic.
Uses: dandruff, mouthwash, cuts, insect bites, candida.

Ylang ylang
Properties: euphoric, aphrodisiac, relaxing.
Uses: depression, tension, high blood pressure, digestive upsets.

all levels. Ayurvedic practitioners often work on the immune system, in order to balance and energize it and keep it strong so that it is able to fight invaders and relieve chronic conditions. There are seven main constitutional types, and once yours is established, you are given a set of guidelines to follow, which add up to an individually prepared plan for physical, mental and spiritual maintenance. Every Ayurvedic programme is completely different and tailored to the individual. There is no one treatment that works for an ailment in every person.

Treats: Ayurvedic medicine can, in theory, address any type of health problem, and is particularly useful for shifting long-term or chronic conditions. In particular, allergies, digestive disorders, anxiety, depression, headaches, insomnia, respiratory problems, skin problems, stress and high blood pressure respond to it.

BACH FLOWER REMEDIES

Bach flower remedies use the vibrationary essence of flowers to balance the negative emotions which lead to and are symptoms of disease. They are a simple natural method of establishing personal equilibrium and harmony.

They are simple to use and can be taken safely by people of all ages and conditions and will not interfere with any other medication. The main dictum of the theory is to 'treat the patient, not the disease'. Its founder, Dr Edward Bach, believed that there is a crucial relationship between the mental outlook of a person and their physical state. When body and soul become disconnected, there is a fundamental imbalance, which leads to illness, disease, and all manner of health problems. Bach believed that plants can re-establish the link between body and soul, between nature and spirit. He stated that emotions such as guilt, fear, doubt, scepticism, self-disgust and self-condemnation could manifest themselves physically as pain, stress and illness with accompanying negative emotions.

Treats: any emotional or mental condition, which will have, overall, a beneficial effect on all health problems. In particular, stress, digestive disorders, sleep problems and skin problems tend to respond well.

CHINESE HERBALISM

Chinese herbalism is the use of herbs to treat and prevent mental, physical and emotional ill-health. The herbs may be in their raw form or processed into pills, powders, ointments, liquid tonics or teas. They are classified according to their properties, such as 'warming', 'cooling', and their taste. Herbal treatment is intended to nourish the body, strengthening and toning weak and depleted energy. Traditional Chinese diagnostic techniques are used to determine the cause of ill health and 'patterns of disharmony' in the body, and herbs are prescribed to restore harmony to mind, body and emotions. Chinese herbalists aim to treat the person, not the illness, and to encourage prevention rather than cure.

Treats: Chinese herbs can be used for a wide range of ailments including asthma, skin diseases, menstrual problems, neurological disorders, infertility, allergies, arthritis, depression, digestive disturbances and migraine and are effective when used on their own or in conjunction with another therapy such as acupuncture.

CHIROPRACTIC

Chiropractic is a medical practice based on the theory that disease results from a disruption of nerve function. This interference is thought to stem primarily from displaced vertebrae, which chiropractors massage and manipulate in order to relieve pressure on nerves. When bones become misaligned, muscles are thrown into spasm, causing immobility of ligaments and tendons, which in turn prevents the body from functioning properly. As a result, most body systems become impaired, and ill-health and pain result. The body's healthy state is restored by moving the bones and joints back to their correct position.

Treats: all back and neck problems, including those caused by tension, injury and congestion. Menstrual problems, headaches, asthma, pregnancy and post-natal problems, digestive and circulatory disorders, some heart conditions, insomnia, and constipation may also be resolved.

HEALING

Over recent decades, healing, also called 'spiritual healing', has finally lost its mystical, magical associations to become one of the most important and popular means of treatment available today. The scientific theory behind healing is still confused, and there are two main schools of thought. Some healers believe that a patient's brainwaves are stimulated during the healing and that it is these waves that cause the healing process to take place, smoothing out imbalances within the body that might cause disease. Most healers, however, believe that they have been given a power that allows them to speed up the body's natural process of healing. Spiritual healing provides the energy required to balance our bodies, minds and spirits, and unblock the healing mechanism.

Treats: healing is used for many conditions, in particular, stress and associated symptoms. It is excellent for emotional disorders, musculo-skeletal disorders, serious medical conditions and chronic illnesses. Some people have reported complete cures from terminal illnesses. Healing can be quite dramatic when it works; or it may not work at all.

Steve Magan
✿ *I have to say that I was very sceptical about homeopathy, but having taken St Johns wort for stress, I changed my mind – it really does work.*

HOMEOPATHY

Homeopathy is a complete system of medicine based on the law of similars – like is cured by like, which means that a substance that produces symptoms in a healthy person would cure those same symptoms when they were caused by illness. Homeopathy is a holistic form of medicine which aims to help the body heal itself. It works for both acute (short-term) illnesses and chronic (long-term) ailments and is concerned as much with preventing illness as it is with treatment. It is the opposite of conventional medicine, which treats illness with an antidote rather than a similar. In conventional medicine, hayfever would be treated by suppressing the symptoms with drugs, such as antihistamines, to stop the itching eyes, running nose and coughing. A homeopath would treat hayfever by introducing minute quantities of allergens which would encourage the body's immune response, and allow it to heal itself.

Homeopathic remedies contain infinitesimal amounts of the original substance diluted in a base. The higher the dilution (and the less of the substance present) the stronger the remedy. In the box opposite we recommend dosages of 6c (dilutions) and 30c. Higher dosages such as 200c are best prescribed by experts.

The remedies are prescribed for the person, not just the disease, and a remedy is not homeopathic because it is prescribed by a homeopath but because it matches exactly the condition of the patient. The choice of remedies is extremely complex, and every aspect of the individual will be taken into consideration before a prescription is made. A homeopath will consider your personal life, habits, emotions, diet, exercise, sleeping patterns, complexion, appetite, moods, posture, environment, weather, libido and many other aspects, and the symptoms themselves are broken down and analysed carefully. The character of the symptoms is as important as the symptoms themselves, as is the constitution of the person experiencing them. Three people experiencing joint pain are likely to require three different remedies.

Treats: homeopathy can conceivably treat any condition, because it addresses every body system. It can be used in some emergency situations, like shock or injury, when it offers remedies to encourage healing and address the problem while you wait for conventional medical help. It addresses emotional conditions, such as panic, anxiety and fear, and most physical conditions.

HYPNOTHERAPY
The British Medical Association have tentatively defined hypnosis in part as 'a temporary condition of altered attention in the subject that may be induced by another person' but there is still much to be understood about it. Although the condition resembles normal sleep, scientists have found that the brain wave patterns of hypnotized subjects are much closer to the patterns of deep relaxation. Hypnosis is a tool for reaching and dealing with problems of the mind and body using a state of mental relaxation in which the patient is open to suggestion. In the hypnotized state, emotional problems can be addressed and resolved, and body functions can be improved to restore normal activity. There is evidence that hormonal problems, respiration, heart rate, circulation and digestive activity can be influenced by hypnosis, and many people find they can cut off completely from sensations of pain.

Treats: hypnotherapy is especially useful in the treatment of behavioural and habitual difficulties, such as smoking, eating disorders and phobias. Other conditions treated include arthritis, asthma, digestive troubles, eczema, insomnia, migraine, stress and many childhood problems such as colic, bed-wetting and hyperactivity. It is very good for chronic pain, such as sciatica and headaches. Some cancers respond to treatment.

MASSAGE
Massage is probably the oldest therapy known to man. Massage involves taking into account a person's whole being – their physical, mental and emotional make-up. It aims to create and maintain the best possible health for the patient by relaxing, stimulating and invigorating mind and body, according to specific needs. Physically, it is aimed at improving the circulation and muscular and nervous systems, also helping the body to assimilate food and get rid of waste products. The most common and effective use of massage is to relax the body and mind and to relieve the strains and tensions of daily life (see p. 48). On its simplest level, it can ease all kinds of pain, and mentally it can have calming and soothing effects. It can also stimulate and revitalize.

Treats: massage can treat many complaints, but it is particularly good for stress and stress-related conditions such as tension, anxiety and headaches, insomnia, depression, circulation problems. It is also good for helping aching and

TOP HOMEOPATHIC REMEDIES

The following homeopathic remedies are perfect for a home first-aid box, and will treat many common health problems and emergencies. When using remember to take only one remedy at a time, don't touch the remedies (empty them on to a teaspoon and put under the tongue), avoid acoholic drinks, cigarettes, spicy or minty foods which will interfere with the healing action, try to take at least 30 minutes after eating, or else first rinse your mouth out with water. Store the remedies in a cool, dark place in a tightly closed bottle away from strong smells.

Arnica
6c or 30c for shock after injury and bruising, cramp, burns, stings, nose bleed, sprains, strained or torn muscles, eczema, boils and bedwetting in children.

Apis
30c for insect stings that are hot and swollen, cystitis, hives, oedema, arthritis, allergic reactions in eyes, throat and mouth. (Avoid during pregnancy.)

Bryonia
30c for swollen painful joints, swollen painful breasts, heat exhaustion, bursting headache and nausea, screaming colicky babies, colds and flu.

Cantharis
6c or 30c for burns, scalds and blisters, cystitis, burning diarrhoea, any burning or stinging sensation.

Euphrasia
6c for conjunctivitis, eye strain or foreign bodies in the eyes, hayfever where the eyes are mainly affected, bursting headaches, constipation.

Glonoin
30c for heat exhaustion, bursting headache, hot flushes.

Hypericum
30c for burns and sunburn, small cuts or grazes, insect bites.

Ledum
6c for a painful black eye, stiffness in the joints, cold-weather complexion; prevents infection.

Nux vomica
6c for travel sickness and nausea with a headache, digestive problems, heavy periods, hangover, morning sickness, cystitis, labour pains.

Phosphate
6c for nose bleeds caused by severe blowing.

Rhus tox
6c for red, swollen, itchy blisters, nappy rash, painful stiff muscles, cramp, rheumatic or arthritic pain that is eased by moving.

Ruta grav
6c for pain and stiffness in pulled muscles, eye strain, rheumatism, deep aching pain in bones and muscles, sciatica.

Silica
6c for splinters that could cause infection, migraine, recurrent colds and infections, spots, weak nails, slow-to-heal fractures.

Tabacum
6c for travel sickness, nausea, vomiting, faintness, dizziness and anxiety.

Urtica
6c for stinging burns, scalds and allergic skin, insect stings, cystitis and hives.

strained muscles, arthritis, rheumatism and sciatica. People with digestive disorders, such as irritable bowel syndrome and constipation, also benefit from the treatment.

NATUROPATHY

Naturopathy is, like ayurveda, more than just a therapy; it is a philosophy for living which involves a health plan and lifestyle changes. It is based on the belief that the body has the ability to heal itself when free of the toxins that are accumulated through poor lifestyle habits. Naturopathy stimulates the body's natural defences and promotes an equilibrium that allows it to function properly and effectively. Naturopaths believe that getting ill is natural and that methods of cure should follow the same natural principles. Symptoms of illness should be encouraged to come out and the body encouraged to resist the invaders and find its proper balance.

Naturopathic treatments include: breathing, hydrotherapy (the use of water to promote healing), baths, douches, enemas, colonic irrigation, diet, fasting, osteopathy and homeopathy.

Treats: naturopathy can help with a wide range of acute and chronic problems such as anaemia, allergies, arthritis, circulation disorders, constipation, cystitis, eczema and other skin diseases, hangovers, irritable bowel syndrome, migraine, pre-menstrual syndrome, ulcers and varicose veins.

TOP HERBAL REMEDIES

These herbs can be used in a variety of forms, depending on the condition you are trying to treat. Use as a compress, as tablets (only take the recommended dosage), teas, creams and many other forms. Have a look around your local healthfood shop – you'll find most of them available. They can, of course, be used fresh, in cooking.

Angelica
Uses: coughs, rheumatic pain, travel sickness, fever, pleurisy, nervousness.

Basil
Uses: insect bites, vomiting, constipation, nervous complaints.

Bay
Uses: rheumatism, fever, bruises and sprains.

Calendula
Uses: for cuts, bruises, grazes and minor skin problems.

Chamomile
Uses: fever, nervous conditions, swelling, sores, fatigue, digestive complaints.

Comfrey
Uses: diarrhoea, stomach ulcers, bleeding gums, period problems, bruises, bites, sores, lung problems, whooping cough, broken bones.

Echinacea
Uses: fighting infection and warding off colds, flu and sore throats. Boosts the immune system while acting as a natural antibiotic.

Elder
Uses: measles, bronchial problems, scarlet fever, colds, skin complaints.

Garlic
Uses: coughs and colds, thrush, wounds, bites, stings, infections, catarrh, high blood cholesterol, high blood pressure.

Ginger
Uses: indigestion and wind, circulatory disorders, arthritis, morning sickness and travel sickness.

Lavender
Uses: relieves stress and promotes relaxation; treats stress and related disorders, insomnia, headaches, infection.

Lime blossom
Uses: tension headaches and the effects of stress, including insomnia.

NUTRITIONAL THERAPY

Nutritional therapy is the therapeutic use of diet to treat and prevent illness, and to restore the body to its natural, healthy equilibrium. Food has always been used for its medicinal effects and we now know that a varied diet, rich in natural ingredients, is essential for good health. Nutritional therapy is based on the belief that each part of the body is made of elements which were once the nutritional elements of food. The idea is that health problems crop up when one of the nutritional links is weak, or missing, and a nutritional therapist will decide how it can be put back in place, using nutrition and knowledge of the body. A healthy body is strong and resistant to illness, and while addressing the symptoms of one illness, by providing overall nutrition, very often other unrelated conditions will be cured. Nutritional therapy involves the use of the elements of nutrition (that is, a balanced diet), perhaps supplemented with vitamins, minerals, amino acids or essential fatty acids, to balance

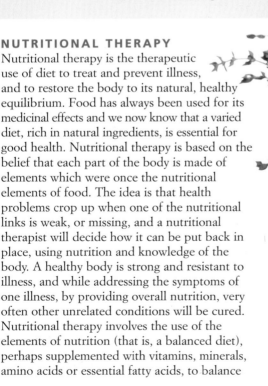

Marjoram
Uses: diarrhoea, flatulence, coughs, cramps, colic, rheumatism, sprains, inflammation, sore throats, bruising.

Meadowsweet
Uses: pain relief and acid indigestion.

Mint
Uses: headaches, insomnia, nervousness, coughs, migraine, flatulence, abdominal aches.

Parsley
Uses: rheumatism, cystitis, insect bites, asthma, stings, urinary ailments, coughs.

Peppermint
Uses: indigestion, flatulence, headaches and colds.

Rosemary
Uses: circulatory disorders, stomach-ache and bruises, headaches and migraine, exhaustion.

Sage
Uses: gastritis, diarrhoea, throat problems, nervousness.

Thyme
Uses: coughs and colds, sore throat, catarrh, whooping cough, headaches, diarrhoea, rheumatism, bruises.

Valerian
Uses: flatulence, nervous headache, insomnia, stress, tension.

any slight deficiencies. The therapeutic use of other nutritional supplements can help to deal with specific health conditions.

Treats: most conditions, in particular, anxiety, arthritis, asthma, depression, digestive disorders, eczema, headaches, herpes, high blood pressure, hormone problems, PMS, osteoporosis, pregnancy problems, reduced immunities, skin problems, stress and viruses. Most importantly, nutritional therapy is preventative.

OSTEOPATHY

Osteopathy is a therapy based on manipulation of bones and muscles. Osteopaths maintain that the normal body produces forces necessarily to fight disease and that most ailments are due to the misalignment of bones and other faulty conditions of the muscle tissue and cartilage. When the spine and skeleton are misaligned, organs malfunction and blood and lymphatic fluid are not able to circulate properly. By

restoring balance and correcting any lesions or misalignment, blood can flow smoothly to the organs, the nervous system is able to function properly, and the lymphatic system is free of any stagnation that can cause toxins to build up. Digestion, respiration and every other body function will be improved as a result of treatment.

Cranial osteopathy involves gently massaging the bones and muscles of the cranium (skull) in order to improve the flow of cerebro-spinal fluid, which bathes the nervous system. The release of tension will affect functions throughout the body.

Treats: back and neck troubles, musculo-skeletal pain, circulation, breathing problems, depression, digestive disorders, constipation, migraine, fatigue, inflammation, joint pain, nausea, neuralgia, sciatica, some skin problems, menstrual and pre-menstrual disorders, stress and eczema. Energy and well-being will be restored to optimum levels.

REFLEXOLOGY

Reflexology involves stimulating, massaging and applying pressure to points on the hands and feet which correspond to various systems and organs throughout the body to stimulate its own healing system. These points are called 'reflex points', and each one corresponds to a different body part or function. Reflexologists believe that applying pressure to these reflex points can improve the health of the body and mind. Depending on the points chosen, reflexology can be used to ease tension, reduce inflammation, relieve congestion, improve circulation and eliminate toxins from the body. Like most other complementary therapists, reflexologists do not claim to cure anything, rather they aim to stimulate the body to heal itself. They do this by working on the physical body to stimulate the healing at physical, mental and emotional levels.

Treats: reflexology is an excellent whole-body system and can be used both to prevent illness and to encourage the body to heal. It is particularly useful for stress and related disorders, emotional disorders, digestive problems, circulatory disorders, menstrual problems, insomnia, fatigue, and most chronic and acute illnesses.

WESTERN HERBALISM

Herbalism is probably the oldest form of recorded medicine, and Western herbalism combines the ancient teachings of the East with indigenous traditions and folk remedies, complemented by modern-day scientific study. Herbalism is the use of plants as medicines to restore and maintain health by keeping the body in balance. It relies on the specific qualities of individual plants to stimulate our own healing system and restore health. Like most holistic practitioners, herbalists believe that we all possess healing energy which they call the 'vital force'. This vital force works constantly to maintain our holistic health – that is, health on spiritual, physical and emotional levels.

Herbal remedies are prescribed to support the affected body systems in their fight against disease. The purpose of the herbs, therefore, is not only to alleviate disease, but also to prevent it recurring, to detoxify the system of poisons that can cause disease and to support the immune system and maintain balance.

Treats: Western herbal medicine treats the same range of conditions that conventional medicine treats. However, in medical emergencies, such as serious injury, acute illness involving the organs or skeleton, or in cases of serious infection or disease, you must always seek urgent conventional medical attention. Western herbalism is particularly good for longer-term, chronic conditions such as allergies, asthma, cystitis, depression, digestive disorders, neuralgia, menstrual problems, respiratory problems, skin problems, stress and viral infections.

YOGA

Yoga is a system of spiritual, mental and physical training. The underlying philosophy stresses the influence of mind over body and holds that mental and spiritual development are necessary to reinforce the benefits that the physical exercises bring (see p. 50). The ancient teachers of yoga worked out some of their postures through watching the movements of animals, which seem to move and relax so much more effectively than humans. The postures are designed to promote flexibility and controlled relaxation. The movements are done slowly and the postures held for a minute or more to build up strength as well as awareness of the body and its tensions and patterns of behaviour. Breathing also plays an important part in yoga (see p. 50), as breath, according to yoga philosophy, embodies our 'prana', or life force.

Treats: anyone can benefit from yoga, and it will help all body systems return to their natural working order. In particular, it treats any type of stress-related problem such as anxiety, high blood pressure, circulation and heart problems, backache, asthma, digestive problems such as irritable bowel syndrome (IBS), fatigue, arthritis, rheumatism and depression.

DIY REFLEXOLOGY

To give yourself a reflexology treatment, sit comfortably with your bare right foot resting on your left leg. Hold your foot with your left hand and work on it with your right. Change position to work on your left foot.

When you work on a specific area, repeat at least three times and when pressing a point hold for about 30 seconds. Repeat the treatment until symptoms subside, but be careful not to overdo it. Begin every treatment by working all over the foot, giving special emphasis to specific reflex points. It might be helpful to have a map of the feet, indicating the reflex points for various parts of the body. Here are some easy treatments for common ailments:

Headaches: massage around the big toe, which relates to the head and neck area.

Indigestion: On the left foot, massage around the centre, just below the ball of the foot, which relaxes to the stomach and pancreas.

Period pains: massage the area on the bottom of the heel of both feet.

Anxiety: begin by stroking all over the foot. Then press the pad of your thumb into the solar plexus, the kidney and the adrenal gland reflexes (which can be found on the centre of the left foot, below the ball of the foot), covering the area from side to side. Finish by stroking all over the foot.

Colds: work the head area (big toes). Then work with your thumb on the affected areas such as the nose, throat and chest, which can be found along the base of all the toes on both feet. If you also have a temperature, work on the pituitary gland reflex, which is found on the big toes of both feet.

Insomnia: work all over the foot, giving special attention to the head area (big toes). Press on the solar plexus, which sits in the centre of the left foot, just below the ball of the foot. Finish by gently stroking the tops of your feet from the toes up towards the ankle.

Stress relief: begin by stroking both feet to relax yourself. Then massage over the head reflexes (big toes), across the shoulders (down the outside of the balls of the feet) and across the balls of the feet, just below the toes. Press the solar plexus (which sits in the centre of the left foot, just below the ball of the foot) and the adrenal reflexes (on the inside of the feet, about halfway down) and release, repeating a number of times.

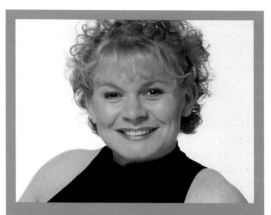

> MY NATURAL FAVOURITES

1. My nana always made my mum have a tablespoon of fish oil once a day. Mum passed it on to me and I even heard her say recently that she can feel her joints are more stiff and achy on the days she doesn't take her supplement. To avoid creaky joints, get lubricated with some cod liver oil.

2. After running my first London Marathon this year, my whole body felt swollen and stiff the morning after so I took some arnica tablets. I really advocate the use of arnica to combat swelling and/or bruising. It works a treat.

3. If I feel panicky and stressed I have four drops of Bach's rescue remedy in water. Whether it's psychological or not, it seems to calm me down.

4. At the first sign of a cold or flu I reach for the echinacea. I add about 15 drops to a glass of water. It can strengthen a weakened immune system and I'm sure, by taking it, my colds never develop as badly as if I hadn't.

5. I take grapefruit seed extract – about 15 drops a day in a glass of water. I do so much rushing around that I can run myself into the ground and the grapefruit seed extract is my insurance policy, keeping my immune system topped up with a natural aid.

MASSAGE OILS

STIMULATING MASSAGE OIL
100 ml/4 oz grapeseed oil
4 ml/1 tsp wheatgerm oil
5 drops cajuput
5 drops peppermint essential oil
Blend together and use sparingly.

RELAXING MASSAGE OIL
100 m1/4 oz grapeseed oil
15 ml/1 tbsp wheatgerm oil
5 drops neroli
5 drops sandalwood essential oil
Blend together and use sparingly.

7. Glenda's top ten health tips

1

Drink water – still mineral water is best, but plain tap water will do. Drink at least one and a half litres a day (six to eight glasses); it will cleanse your system, keep you hydrated, keep your skin clear, combat water retention, help you keep a clear head and refresh you.

2

I used to suffer very badly from PMS, both abdominal pain and bad moods. Taking 500 mg of evening primrose oil daily changed my life and almost eradicated PMS. My time of the month is just about bearable now so I recommend it.

3

Try to exercise at least three times a week. Exercise is so good for you, it energizes you, tones up your muscles, makes your heart stronger, your lungs more efficient, builds your bone density, gets rid of your cellulite, de-stresses you... the list is endless, but I must not forget to mention those brain chemicals that make you happy – endorphins. Endorphins are released into the bloodstream as you work out, so it's official: exercise will give you a buzz and make you feel better than before you pulled your trainers on. Get working out!

4

Think positively. I have spent years feeling self-conscious about my body and wishing I looked thinner and more beautiful. I taught myself to think positively and feel healthier and happier for it. Life is too short to worry and get depressed about things that you just can't change – I'm afraid I will never be size 10. Try to be happy with who you are and how you look. Having inner confidence makes you sparkle in the eyes of others, plus you won't worry so much, so your stress levels will be lower and therefore you will be healthier too.

5

By all means take a multivitamin and mineral supplement if you lead a really busy life and don't get a chance to eat fresh fruit and vegetables every day. The health tip is to remember that it is just a supplement, not a replacement. Try whenever you can to eat fresh fruit and vegetables – the body is more likely to absorb vitamins and minerals from natural produce than a refined pill. Plus fruit and veg give you added fibre and they are yummy.

6

You'll like this one – remember to rest. In today's hectic world it is often the aspect of overall good health that we miss out. Rest and relaxation are essential to restore both mind and body. I have had times in the past when I have not taken five minutes out each day to clear my mind and chill out. This used to result in me getting so tense and tired that I got ratty with people, couldn't think straight or cope with the easiest of tasks. Just five minutes sitting in your garden, listening to music or reading a book or magazine relaxes the mind, de-stresses the body and, I've found, makes it much easier to go back to the job in hand, smiling, revved and able to do it three times quicker (thus saving myself time, effort and stress in the long run).

7

If you really can't face the idea of a gym, an aerobics class or any type of team sport, please try to follow this tip. Don't take the lift, use the stairs, walk to the corner shop, don't jump in the car, or even do a few stretching exercises before getting in the shower in the morning – it'll help wake you up. If the weather is nice outside, get yourself out for a stroll – even if it is in your lunch break or walking to meet the kids from school rather than driving. Do it! It will revitalize you, tone up your muscles, burn unwanted fat and improve your fitness, as well as being great for your lungs and heart.

8

My mum had a very high cholesterol reading when she went for a 'well woman' check-up at the doctor's a couple of years ago. She really didn't fancy the thought of all her arteries getting slowly clogged, her blood pressure going up and the risk of heart disease, so she went on a low-fat diet. Now any of you who have seen my video, *Fit, Fresh and Funky*, know how slim and fantastic she looks. She has lost loads of weight simply by eating the correct food. Please try to cut down on margarine and butter (read the chapter on nutrition for more detailed information). Trust my mum and me, you will lose weight and your body will be healthier.

9

If you find it difficult to unwind, relax or sleep, lavender is the essential oil for you. I swear by it. A couple of drops in the bath will de-stress you after a busy day. Put some in an incense burner and fill your room with a relaxing aroma to smooth out your stresses and strains. Or, alternatively, if you find it hard to fall asleep at night, a couple of drops on your pillow will mean you won't have to resort to counting sheep again. It works for me.

10

Don't get too hung up or obsessive about any of this – believe me, I don't! Use this book as a guide, not a bible. Just remember, everything in moderation. My aim is not to preach to you. You will enjoy life more if you live it to the full – and having a little bit of what you fancy does you good. If you get home from work stressed out, have a glass of wine; it will relax you and lower your blood pressure too. It's exactly what I do. I just don't take it to excess – not too often anyway.

Useful addresses

Acupuncture

The British Acupuncture
Council
Park House
106–108 Latimer Road
London W10 6RE

Alexander Technique

Society of Teachers of the
Alexander Technique
20 London House
266 Fulham Road
London SW10 9EL

Aromatherapy

Aromatherapy Organisations
Council
3 Latymer Close
Braybrooke
Market Harborough
Leicester LE16 8LN

International Federation of
Aromatherapists
Stamford House
2–4 Chiswick High Road
London W4 1TH

Ayurveda

Ayurvedic Medical Association
UK
The Hale Clinic
7 Park Crescent
London W1N 3HE

Ayurvedic Company of Great
Britain
50 Penywern Road
London SW5 9XS

Bach Flower Remedies

The Bach Centre
Mount Vernon
Sotwell, Wallingford
Oxfordshire OX10 9PZ

Chinese Herbalism

The Register of Chinese Herbal
Medicine (RCHM)
PO Box 400
Wembley
Middlesex HA9 9NZ

Chiropractic

The British Chiropractic
Association
Equity House
29 Whitley Street
Reading RG2 0EG

Healing

Association for Therapeutic
Healers
Flat 5
54–56 Neal Street
Covent Garden
London WC2

The National Federation of
Spiritual Healers (NFSH)
Old Manor Farm Studio
Church Street
Sunbury-on-Thames
Middlesex TW16 6RG

Herbalism

National Institute of Medical
Herbalists
56 Longbrooke Street
Exeter EX4 8HA

The General Council and
Register of Consultant
Herbalists
18 Sussex Square
Brighton
East Sussex BN2 5AA

Homeopathy

The British Homeopathic
Association
27A Devonshire Street
London WC1N 1RJ

Society of Homeopaths
2 Artizan Road
Northampton NN1 4HU

Hypnotherapy

British Hypnotherapy
Association
67 Upper Berkeley Street
London W1H 7DH

National Register of
Hypnotherapists and
Psychotherapists
12 Cross Street
Nelson
Lancs
BB9 7EN

Massage

The British Massage Therapy
Council
Greenbank House
65A Adelphi Street
Preston PR1 7BH

Index

Bold type indicates main sections